LOVER
EXORCIST
CRITIC

LOVER
EXORCIST
CRITIC
Understanding
Depth Psychotherapy

Alan Michael Karbelnig

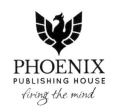

PHOENIX
PUBLISHING HOUSE
firing the mind

First published in 2024 by
Phoenix Publishing House Ltd
62 Bucknell Road
Bicester
Oxfordshire OX26 2DS

British Library Cataloguing in Publication Data

A C.I.P. for this book is available from the British Library

ISBN-13: 978-1-800131-96-5

Typeset by Medlar Publishing Solutions Pvt Ltd, India

www.firingthemind.com

To

Amy, the love of my life,

and

To

our daughters, Misha and Natalie,
their husbands, Jim and Tom,
and our angelic grandchild, Naomi.

Contents

Acknowledgments

Within a few years of my first clinical psychology internship in 1979, watching senior psychoanalytic scholars struggle to define psychoanalysis troubled me. Professors and supervisors alike wrestled with categorizing the subject they taught—an unbearable irony. After obtaining extensive education and experience myself, and masochistically earning the status of Training and Supervising Psychoanalyst (recognized by the American and International Psychoanalytic Associations), I took to tackling the problem myself. The metaphors of lover, exorcist, and critic formed the first few images of a new unique organizational system. Explaining the meaning of these analogies in this book—more than ten years in the making—represents a major step toward explaining, in understandable terms, precisely how *depth psychotherapy* works.

As noted in greater detail in the Preface to *Lover, Exorcist, Critic: Understanding Depth Psychotherapy* (LEC), the phrase *depth psychotherapy* covers a wide range of psychoanalytic psychotherapies. These include formal psychoanalysis itself—defined as patients lying prone on a couch for psychoanalytic sessions held minimally four times per week. Even in the early days of my career, these designations struck me as absurd. Why constrict a two-person, interpersonal transformational experience by requiring a specific number of sessions? And why insist upon the couch? Sigmund Freud, who invented psychoanalysis as the nineteenth century transitioned into the twentieth, is responsible for these traditions. He used the couch, and he required patients to consult him six sessions per week. Interestingly, Freud used the term *Monday crust* to describe resistances encountered in patients who, because he took that one day off, were more defensive. The 48-hour break partially sealed up, and therefore limited his access to, patients' unconscious wounds. Every single aspect of the world, from physics to neuropsychology, from technology to globalization, has exponentially evolved since then. We now live in a technology-contaminated, hyper-capitalist, and de-humanized 21st century. Contemporary psychoanalytic approaches, providing a rare and crucial service by privileging individual human subjectivity, need not comport to standards established while Queen Victoria still reigned.

As such, depth psychotherapy cannot and should not be arbitrarily associated with session frequency or use of the couch. Responsibility for these decisions belongs, instead, to each unique psychoanalyst–patient dyad. In the ensuing pages, I expand upon my definition of depth psychotherapy, suggesting it contains three universal, basic components: *framing, presence,* and *engagement.* I also introduce four foundational phenomena—the unconscious and its manifestations in the transference, repetition compulsion, and dreams (as well as other signifiers of the unconscious mind). As I explain in great detail, these unite even widely divergent psychoanalytic approaches and need not require archaic practices, like patients lying prone on a couch, to be effective.

I owe thanks to many individuals, including some who offered ideas in the earliest days of my working on this project. David Impastato, Nora Smith, Dana Amarisa, and Natalie Abeles offered editorial and conceptual advice from the get-go. Enrico Gnaulati, another scholarly friend and colleague, has four published books; we meet up often to have fun, discuss ideas, and provide needed encouragement for our writing projects. Revealing the true meaning of oedipal conflicts, some of my motivation resulted from competitive urges triggered by Enrico's publishing success. David Impastato and I enjoy a rare male friendship lasting well over forty years. During a one-year period, our friendship almost ended when he offered to edit a few chapters without compensation.

The tension reached nearly fisticuff heights when I (foolishly) disregarded many of his suggestions. My other "best friend," David Wolff, also offered much-needed emotional support and helpful ideas. When and if I fall into dementia, I shall appreciate having two close friends sharing the same name. Easy to remember.

Since the editing misadventure with David Impastato, and for many years now, Andrea Rosas Howe has provided invaluable editing and copyreading assistance to me. Although not in the field, Andrea understands the meaning of the lover, the exorcist, and the critic more than many psychoanalytic professionals. Her editorial services included submitting the book proposal to publishing houses, offering ideas for cover art, managing my weekly newsletter (titled "Journeys to the Unconscious Mind"), and more. She not only reviewed the *LEC* manuscript with an eye on grammar, structure, and continuity, but she also made stylistic suggestions like moving paragraphs or sections to improve the reader experience. Her husband, Josh Howe, deserves a shout-out as well. He manages my website and all things digital and meta-universal.

I owe a debt of thanks to other professionals involved in the publication of this work. Special thanks to Kate Pearce of Phoenix Publishing, who triggered near-euphoria in me when her July 25, 2022, email pronounced:

> The editorial board unanimously agrees your book fits perfectly into the Phoenix list and you bring a fresh understanding to depth psychotherapy that will appeal widely. The book is well-written, engaging, and the use of the three case studies interwoven throughout the book alongside theory works brilliantly.

I may print these sentences, frame them, and hang them on a wall next to my lonely writing desk. Her acknowledgment of the metaphors I propose for depth psychotherapy means the world to me; the compliment about writing quality didn't hurt. Along similar lines, I offer thanks to Mark Kerr of Rowman and Littlefield and Alexis O'Brien of Taylor & Francis, who passed on *LEC*. I appreciate their care in reviewing the work and suggesting other publishing houses. Regarding other professionals, I use my intellectual property attorney, Jim Duda, Esq., of Bulkley, Richardson and Gelinas, LLP in Springfield, Massachusetts, to impress colleagues. You can imagine the line, right? "I'll have to run this by my attorney, etc."

Truth be told, Jim and I have been close friends since we were roommates before the end of the last century. In a story I fit into a novel-in-process titled *The Radioactive Psychoanalyst: Mad, Bad, and Dangerous to Know*, Jim snuck into a Santa Monica, California house I rented during my undergraduate years. We could live cheaply by sharing rooms in a four-bedroom house not far from UCLA. While preparing to move in and lacking a housekey, Jim pried open a window and stuck his head and neck inside. In that most vulnerable of bodily positions, he encountered the smartest-dog-ever, a 22-lb mixed-breed dog named Daisy. Lucky for him, not to mention his profession, Jim's a smooth talker. Daisy growled for a few minutes. Jim complimented her on her beauty and wit. Within seconds, Daisy's tail began wagging. She allowed him to wriggle his body the rest of the way into the house unharmed.

A few depth psychotherapists, both immersed in the Jungian school, helped me personally over the decade I worked on the book. Michael Gellert and Cyndy Rothe, the latter whom I still consult once a week, encourages immersion in *being*—almost applying a Buddhist perspective. Our work reminds me of Penn's struggles. Depth psychotherapy offers a crucible for self-reflection unavailable in any other medium. Friendships, even the most intimate, remain understandably constricted by censorship. Competent depth psychotherapy assists in identifying one's authentic voice. Both Michael and Cydny helped me to bring the truest possible articulation to *LEC*. I also send a shout-out to Alice Cheng, another dear person who similarly has helped me on my personal journey.

I have many colleagues who I also consider friends. They offered emotional support, as well as occasional ideas, as I stumbled through creating and editing this manuscript. Jon Mills, a Canadian philosopher and psychologist, provided remarkable help. Our friendship blossomed when I shared the rejection of one of my articles by the journal *Psychoanalytic Dialogues*. The friendship was instantly forged, and it thrives to this day. Jon almost insisted I continue working on *LEC*, pointing out how scholars enjoy greater freedom when writing books as opposed to articles. Jon reviewed the book proposal, suggested publishers he knew, and connected me with a few of his own contacts.

I send special thanks to Helen Yee, Ron Novotny, Bobbi O'Brien, Stuart Kirschbaum, Debbie Kirschbaum, Linda Kallan, James Goodwin, Bob Ozwoeld, Robin Lewis, Steve Karbelnig, David Levy, and Sam Karbelnig—friends and family alike—who supported me personally. In my view, we're all family now. Peiyi He, Mona Kumar, Deborah Peters, Ryan Witherspoon, and Joy Merritt showed great excitement about my ideas. They, too, provided yet another emotional foundation for facilitating my creation and ultimate completion of this work. Most writers thank a supreme being, but my belief system in that regard remains in process. I'm not sure we can consider it intelligent, but, for sure, our lives exist in a boundless context enshrouded in mystery. Atheism requires a leap of faith I cannot take. To avoid tribalism, I often switch metaphors. Of late, I prefer *Shiva*, the Hindu god of the dance, of creation and destruction. Ergo, thank you, *Shiva*, for helping this work come into existence.

The endless cliches about love meaning everything cannot be overstated. My family's love, and tolerance for my long periods of writing, allowed me to ultimately finish *LEC*. These include my loving wife of forty years, Amy, our daughters, Misha and Natalie, and their husbands, Jim and Tom. I send a special nod to my three-year-old granddaughter, Naomi. With a single, innocent smile, she evokes both conflict and motivation: conflict over writing versus playing with her, and motivation to create a work that she herself might enjoy decades from now.

About the author

Dr. Alan Karbelnig practices psychoanalysis, psychoanalytic psychotherapy, and couples therapy in Pasadena, California. He earned two PhDs, one in Counseling Psychology from the University of Southern California (USC) in 1986, and a second in Psychoanalysis from the New Center for Psychoanalysis (NCP) in 1996. Later, he was Certified in Psychoanalysis by the American Psychoanalytic Association, which also bestowed him with the status of a Supervising and Training Psychoanalyst. Dr. Karbelnig is also Board Certified in Forensic Psychology by the American Board of Professional Psychology. He founded, serves on the Board of Directors of, and teaches at Rose City Center—a not-for-profit psychoanalytic psychotherapy clinic serving the economically disadvantaged in California. An award-winning teacher, Dr. Karbelnig lectures locally, nationally, and internationally, including in Beijing, China, and in Delhi and Ahmedabad, India and Tel Aviv, Israel. He has published twelve scholarly articles and three book chapters. He also writes a weekly Substack newsletter titled, "Journeys into the Unconscious Mind." *Lover, Exorcist, Critic: Understanding Depth Psychotherapists' Work* is his first book.

Preface

Psychoanalysis, subjectivity, and freedom

I was nine years old when my parents first started worrying about me. I felt sullen about my sickly, inferior status. I grew tired of kids teasing me and picking me last for sports games. I became depressed. Later, the painful emotions coalesced, erupting as rage. I slapped a kid twice my size. He beat me up, fracturing three of my ribs. I changed the combination on the bicycle lock of another kid who bullied me. I felt triumphant. His parents rented a truck to get his bike home. I told one of my teachers she "sucked." When she sent me to the principal's office, I refused to speak.

But the final straw was this:

One day I told my mother, "Go to hell!"

The angry, disrespectful remark earned me my first visit to a psychoanalyst—better described by the broader term *depth psychotherapist*. These clinicians focus on deeper, unconscious themes, on dark emotions. I resisted. But my parents forced me. The elderly gentleman, ensconced in a darkened university office lined with mahogany bookshelves, greeted me with a warm smile. He listened to my tales of insecurity, fears, and furies. When he asked me to elaborate, I told him about the kid I slapped, the lock I changed, and the principal I ignored. The psychoanalyst administered a Rorschach Inkblot test. I told him what I saw in the gray, orange, and red images. Although I had been dispatched only for a consultation, I wished I had more time with the kind old man. His words soothed me. I didn't know why, but they did. I felt better after talking to him. A few years later, when my fury bordered on the violent, my parents often referred to the psychoanalyst's conclusion.

"You have tremendous anger," they told me.

I felt rebuked.

They brought me to him for answers.

I already knew *that* answer.

Many years later, having undergone more extensive depth psychotherapy and entered the profession myself, I gained an understanding of my rage and its relation to my early life experiences. The gray-haired, tall psychoanalyst set me on a path to discover how many of my needs had gone unsatisfied, how my passions went unnoticed, and how my parents' neglect, caused, in part, by their busy 1960s lifestyle—enraged me. I *was* a furious boy, adolescent, and young man. But, of course, that lovely psychoanalyst lacked sufficient time to help me to further identify, articulate, and address these primitive feelings.

As I introduce this book about how psychoanalysis or any type of depth psychotherapy works, that cordial man, his friendly demeanor, and his welcoming office come to mind. He definitely helped me transform from an angry teenager into an assertive, opinionated adult. Depth psychotherapy stimulates growth in varied ways—resolving traumatic pain, exploring meaning, releasing untapped talent. In a phrase, it elucidates persons' subjectivities. It expands their awareness of how they perceive self as well as other, initiating waves of interpersonal, social, and even political change.

Writing a half-century after I met the doctor-with-the-inkblots, I believe depth psychotherapy matters more than ever. We live in an era dubbed "post-humanist,"[1] a period psychoanalyst Christopher Bollas calls the "age of bewilderment."[2] We ingest social programming at unprecedented rates. Anything not observable, measurable, weighable, or consumable lacks value. The ideas of agency, autonomy, and even freedom are increasingly marginalized. Christopher Lasch, a contemporary historian and social critic who coined the phrase, "the minimal self," writes:

> Beyond the injunction to "get in touch with your feelings"—a remnant of an earlier "depth" psychology—lies the now-familiar insistence that there is no depth, no desire even, and that the human personality is merely a collection of needs programmed either by biology or by culture.[3]

Depth psychotherapy, a phrase broadly encompassing a wide variety of psychoanalytic or psychodynamic approaches, counters these individuality-constricting social forces. It facilitates exploration of the unconscious mind, including how sociocultural, historical, and other contextual features affect subjective experiences. Psychoanalytic approaches, ranging from the original Freudian, Kleinian, or Jungian ones to the more recently developed object relations, self-psychology, and intersubjective or relational models, share this consciousness-expanding goal.

While psychoanalysts facilitate their transformational processes, patients share what they have barely dared to tell themselves. They tell stories—of triumph and failure, of love and loss, of meaning and nihilism. They explore attitudes—biases, distortions, preferences, and stereotypes. They experience feelings—sadness, shame, guilt, anxiety, loss, terror, and joy. In several scholarly articles,[4] I proposed that psychoanalysts stimulate growth by *framing* their professional relationships, by offering *presence* in the form of empathy or attunement, and by *engaging* their patients in dialogue—conscious and unconscious, verbal and nonverbal. These ways of structured, interpersonal relating alter patients' *internalization* processes, bringing their intrapsychic conversations, and their previously hidden feelings, thoughts, attitudes, and behaviors, into the light of day.

Internalization processes exist on a continuum ranging from the conscious, like the quiet internal conversations you know about, to dissociated mental content, like disavowed conflicts or deficits (unmet need states), to actual, concretized unconscious structures such as the superego or "dynamic structures."[5] (Proposed by psychoanalyst Ronald Fairbairn, dynamic structures consist of parts of self (or ego) linked to internal representations of other; they exist in the unconscious and propel an inner drama influencing our relationships and our life path.) Depth psychotherapy uncovers and alters the dynamics of these conscious and unconscious internal conversations. Again, these conversations range from the conscious secrets we tell no one else, through the problematic behaviors we disavow, to those we essentially are blind to—through denial. Denial, as formally understood, signifies the transition into the *actual* unconscious. In the unconscious realm lie any number of phenomena obviously outside of consciousness. They may be described as id, ego, superego, dynamic structures, or, to use Melanie Klein's metaphor for unconscious structure, "unconscious phantasies."[6] Put more simply, psychoanalyst Jacques Lacan reduces psychoanalysis to the process of liberating the *subject*, namely the real, authentic you, from the *ego*, the you created to please your parents, society, and other sociocultural influences.

Although Freud intended to introduce a new, modernist form of medical intervention when he named the profession *psychoanalysis* in 1896, he instead launched what ultimately evolved into a method for illuminating the human *subject*. The radical approach toward self-understanding and transformation began as a method for treating mental disorders. Mostly, these were the hysteric and conversion disorders common at the time. Over time, though, psychoanalysts turned their attention to persons other than those with pathological mental conditions. The two World Wars brought traumatized soldiers and civilians alike to seek their help. During and after the Vietnam War, feminism and civil rights came to a head, European existentialism gained in international popularity, and adherence to religion waned. As a result, persons feeling lost, alienated, or having other problems in living began cascading into psychotherapists' consulting rooms. Depth psychotherapists helped persons deal with tragic losses, with fragile senses of self, or with feelings of loneliness just as frequently as they counseled individuals with anxiety, depression, or psychosis.

We all have unconscious themes, which I prefer to call internal dramas.[7] They prevent us from fully becoming who we are, from enjoying deep, intersubjective intimacy, or from working or playing in ways that are maximally satisfying. As Lacan noted, these dramas serve the falsely accommodating *ego*. They beg for replacing with dramas more reflective of the true, authentic self, the *subject*. These internal dramas restrict personal freedom in myriad ways: Promoting inauthenticity, launching harsh self-criticism, or compulsively repeating destructive patterns, to name but a few. The process of helping patients uncover and alter these internal dramas therefore constitutes an intensely humanistic, freedom-enhancing endeavor. By introducing psychoanalysis as a distinct profession, Freud unwittingly re-kindled the Romantic project, that revolutionary reaction to the Enlightenment, the Industrial Revolution, scientism, and other reductionist forces shaping humanity then and now. He joined the ranks of philosophers, political scientists, and writers such as Kant, Nietzsche, Hegel, Rousseau, Keats, Blake, Wordsworth, Dostoyevsky, Tolstoy, Thoreau, and Whitman. These artists rejected the devaluation of all things that could not be measured, weighed, or quantified. They rebelled against objectification. They privileged the subjective.

These intellectuals influenced broad swaths of humanity.

Psychoanalysts similarly exert influence, but slowly—and one person at a time.

Contemporary culture assaults the unique nature of personal *subjectivity* like never before in human history. The extremely rapid advancement of technology, for example, alters the *experience* of being human, particularly in how we communicate. People spend less time speaking face-to-face. Their use of words, gestures, and touch has lessened. They rarely sit down and talk. They email rather than write. They send texts rather than make calls. As contemporary comedian Aziz Ansari puts it, "What—are you on fire? Quit wasting my time. Text me that shit!"

And more change awaits us. Already, common household items wirelessly connect us to the web. Soon, your refrigerator—rather than your spouse, roommate, or lover—will tell you when groceries need ordering. Your automobile already informs you which parts need replacing. Companies like Tesla automatically download software, spontaneously making some repairs. Your house, apartment, work site, rapid transit vehicles, and more will advise you, in computer-generated-faux-feminine-soothing-voice tones, of their status. One could argue, as did Wittgenstein,[8] that technology frees persons to perform tasks more effectively. It gives them more time to commune with one another. But he died before the invention of Skype, Instagram, Tinder, Facebook, Twitter, TikTok, or YouTube. Ironically, these media, intended to accelerate information and to monetize sociability, only draw persons more deeply inward.

They may well result in us talking *more*.

But we are mostly talking *at* each other.

And, when not in monologue, we are forced to listen. The only silent space exists behind our noise-canceling headphones. Except for such blissful, safe, hidden moments, we are constantly besieged by information. The international media delivers its biased content; the international advertising industry aggressively coerces us. We, in turn, passively cooperate by staring at television sets, computer monitors, or mobile phone screens. On a daily basis, we are exposed to thousands of conflicting new "facts," and to thousands of different brand names. These oppressive, invasive mechanisms of interpersonal influence objectify, stultify, and imprison subjectivity, compromising our capacity to freely think, feel, behave—or even imagine. Humans, once accustomed to living life as experiencing *subjects*, instead exist as consuming *objects*. French philosopher Michel Foucault describes the modern human as an "object of information, never a subject in communication."[9] Many people need help not only to counter their own unconscious dramatic themes, but also to offset the invasive information overload contaminating their capacity to find their authentic selves.

Depth psychotherapy encourages these creative, freedom-loving, self-actualizing forces. In confirmation, Mari Ruti proclaims technology and the mass media promote "conformist yearnings that masquerade as our desire," adding depth psychotherapy seeks, in contrast, to "release the singularity of our being from underneath the Other's oppressive signifiers."[10] Here, Ruti acknowledges the essential role of freedom in the depth psychotherapy process, working as it does to liberate patients from oppression on all fronts—internal and external alike.

When persons feel chronically insecure or inadequate, find themselves trapped in unsatisfying jobs or relationships, or habitually engage in self-defeating habits, they live in a state of self-deception, of internal oppression. Psychoanalysis exposes these dark recesses of human subjectivity. Further, it introduces people to the indoctrination, the lies, and the distortions affecting our perceptions of ourselves, of others, and of the world. Breaking through our internal conversations proves difficult—whether we learned them in childhood or had them imposed on us by contemporary culture. Depth psychotherapy offers arguably the *only* professional service directly intended to reverse self-deception and indoctrination. By enlightening subjectivity, by raising consciousness, depth psychotherapy liberates.

Its mission is *freedom*.

Meanwhile, the global, regressive trend to objectify the human subject marches forward, impacting depth psychotherapy itself. Contemporary culture increasingly mandates empirically based and objectively measurable interventions in educational, medical, and other institutions.[11] Psychotherapies comporting with the renewed emphasis on empiricism, such as cognitive behavioral therapy (CBT), lack an emphasis on personal freedom and autonomy. They provide rapid symptom relief but, by design, avoid uncovering unconscious themes. For example, if a barista at Starbucks becomes depressed, the firm's Employee Assistance Program (EAP) would likely refer him or her for a short-term course of cognitive behavioral therapy. The CBT psychotherapist would strive to reduce the employee's emotional discomfort and return him or her to work as rapidly as possible. Such a therapist would *not* pursue the *meaning* of the emotional discomfort. If the symptom represents a minor adjustment problem, then perhaps no harm has been done. But if, for example, the barista's psychological problem *actually* refers to an underlying, deeper conflict, or betrays unsatisfied authentic needs, then CBT or similar forms of behavioral psychotherapy serves Starbucks rather than the employee. It enhances what Karl Marx called alienation[12] because of the gap between what humans *desire* and what they ultimately *do*. His concept of alienation relates to *wage slavery*. Many of us work in jobs we hate, counting the seconds until our evenings or weekends free us from our oppressive work. Psychotherapies like CBT serve the interests of corporations rather than of individuals. It maintains the status quo. It supports workforces by constricting rather than by expanding subjectivities.

Perhaps precisely because it liberates, psychoanalysis threatens our post-humanist, audit-oriented, global society. Any endeavor daring to explore the ambiguous, shadowy world of human subjectivity risks becoming—irony intended—*subject* to suspicion. You've seen the assault. It's ubiquitous. Although serving as only the messengers, major media conglomerates such as *Time* magazine, *The New York Times*, or *The Wall Street Journal* repeatedly proclaim psychoanalysis' demise. CBT overshadows depth psychotherapy in the curricula of most clinical psychiatry and psychology programs. Formal psychoanalytic training institutes have difficulty filling their classes.[13] If anything, dark sociocultural forces already impacting the field risk the extinction of the depth psychotherapy approaches.

A CBT approach would have literally hurt, rather than helped, that angry boy—me—whose parents delivered him to the gentle psychoanalyst all those years ago. It may have reduced my rage, and helped me adhere to academic demands. However, my continued lack of awareness of what angered me may have stunted my emotional growth. No behavioral intervention would have enlightened and, therefore, empowered me. Even after my parents dropped me off for that first meeting with the psychoanalyst, I remained in hiding for years, unable to discover why I was literally going *mad*. Only later did I work through the tremendous loss and sadness hidden beneath my rage, causing my primitive fury to lessen in strength and to morph into assertion, engagement, and passion. I ultimately explored those feelings with my parents, bringing greater understanding, even closeness, to my relationship with them. Just as it worked to free me, the psychoanalytic process releases persons from shackles inside and out. It helps patients not only experience less pain, but cope more effectively with life's ongoing challenges. It encourages authenticity, allowing lives to be led with fullness and vibrancy.

In *Lover, Exorcist, and Critic*, I seek primarily to *educate* about depth psychotherapy, to explain it, and to demonstrate in vivid detail how the process *really* unfolds. I expect many readers find concepts of the self, the mind, and the soul intriguing. I imagine you either consult psychotherapists or have contemplated doing so. You may have felt mystified, as many do, about how the depth psychotherapy process works. I hope to extend Thomas Szasz'[14] de-mythologizing of depth psychotherapy further, throwing the final dirt on the coffin of the medical model from which it emerged. Unlike Szasz, however, I explain how psychoanalysis includes more than the combination of rhetoric and logic. It also features an intersubjective, inter-emotional, interpersonal, and even inter-biological exchange—way too complex to fit within the confines of any one theoretical model.

This book also promotes a *political* agenda. By offering examples of the freedom-enhancing nature of psychoanalysis, I advocate for greater personal agency and autonomy as vehicles for counteracting this bewildering, post-humanist era of the minimal self. These dehumanizing trends are *dangerous*. They risk putting more of us to sleep, numbing us to the vibrancy of our authentic selves. I warn you, in advance, of the polemical tone necessary to advance the political theme. I also prepare you—although here I might be talking to myself rather than to you—to the ways I expose my own vulnerabilities, and even a few outright errors, in my work with the three fictional patients presented. Enduring shame and guilt as I composed some passages, I nonetheless think an authentic story of how psychoanalysis works must be told. It should make it a more exhilarating read. Franz Kafka wrote to his friend Pollack in 1904:

> I think we ought to read only the kind of books that wound and stab us. If the book we're reading doesn't wake us up with a blow on the head, what are we reading it for? We need the books that affect us like a disaster, that grieve us deeply, like the death of someone we loved more than ourselves, like being banished into forests far from everyone, like a suicide. A book must be the axe for the frozen sea inside us.[15]

Inspired by the great surrealist himself, *Lover, Exorcist, and Critic* discloses many wounds and stabs sustained by patients *and* me. In sharing the discipline with such vulnerability, and by delivering a unique perspective of these three unusual metaphors, the book delivers what the contemporary culture's view of psychoanalysis needs most: a smack to the head.

Notes

1. Wolfe, C. (2010). *What is Posthumanism?* Minneapolis, MN: University of Minneapolis Press.
2. Bollas, C. (2015). Psychoanalysis in the age of bewilderment: on the return of the oppressed. *International Journal of Psychoanalysis*, 96(3): 535–551.

3. Lasch, C. (1984). *The Minimal Self: Psychic Survival in Troubled Times*. New York, NY: Norton, pp. 57–58.

4. Karbelnig, A.M. (2022). Chasing infinity: Why clinical psychoanalysis' future lies in pluralism. *International Journal of Psychoanalysis*, 103(1): 5–25.

5. Fairbairn, W.R.D. (1952). *Psychoanalytic Studies of the Personality*. London: Tavistock, p. 377.

6. Klein, M. (1946). Notes on some schizoid mechanisms. *The International Journal of Psychoanalysis*, 27: 99–110.

7. Karbelnig, A.M. (2020). The theater of the unconscious mind. *Psychoanalytic Psychology*, 37(4): 273–281. https://doi.org/10.1037/pap0000251.

8. Wittgenstein, L. (1958). *Philosophical Investigations*. Third Edition. G.E.M. Anscombe (Trans.). Upper Saddle River, NJ: Prentice-Hall.

9. Foucault, M. (1991). *Discipline and Punish: The Birth of the Prison*. A. Sheridan (Trans). New York, NY: Vintage, p. 200.

10. Ruti, R. (2012). *The Singularity of Being: Lacan and the Immortal Within*. New York, NY: Fordham University Press, p. 49.

11. Strathern, N. (Ed). (2010). *Audit Cultures: Anthropological Studies in Accountability, Ethics, and the Academy*. New York, NY: Routledge, p. 2.

12. Marx, K. (1988). *Economic and Philosophical Manuscripts of 1844*. M. Milligan Trans. New York, NY: Prometheus. (Original work published in 1844.)

13. Schechter K (2014). *Illusions of a Future: Psychoanalysis and the Biopolitics of Desire*. Durham and London: Duke University Press.

14. Szasz, T. (1988). *The Ethics of Psychoanalysis*. Syracuse, NY: Syracuse University Press.

15. Kafka, F. (1959). *Letters to Friends, Family and Editors*. New York, NY: Schocken, p. 16.

CHAPTER 1

A polemical introduction

Despite its helping millions of individual patients and impacting twentieth-century culture en masse, many global citizens still regard psychoanalysis with suspicion. They think it mysterious. When hearing the word *psychoanalysis*, people think of gray-bearded, pipe-smoking, ancient white-male practitioners seated behind patients lying prone on red-felt, Victorian-era couches. These images, nearly a century out of date, urgently need an edit, an update. I offer such a revision—a clear, understandable explanation of the unnecessarily obscure profession. In addition, by examining the common threads binding various psychoanalytic schools, I seek to unify a field in which Freudians still fight with Jungians, Kleinians with Bionians, and so on. Other petty arguments persist. Despite their oft-heated disagreements, psychoanalytic clinicians *actually practice* in more similar than dissimilar ways. They raise consciousness and elucidate subjectivities; they enhance patients' personal autonomy and freedom.

Mahatma Gandhi would have loved the field, most likely because of its less understood emphasis on emancipation. Psychoanalysis promotes Gandhi's *satyagraha*—loyalty to truth. He invented the word from two Sanskrit word fragments—*satya*, loosely translated as "truth," and *graha*, meaning "insistence." Psychoanalysis confronts patients with their true selves, altering images of self *and* other. It liberates them from their egos—representing whom they *think* they are. It illuminates their authentic selves, their lives as human subjects. How? By uncovering hidden thoughts, feelings, and fantasies; identifying recurring problematic themes; and studying the dynamics of the psychoanalytic relationship itself. Jonathan Shedler, a contemporary scholar devoted to studying depth psychotherapy's effectiveness, succinctly identifies the process as "exploring those aspects of self that are not fully known, especially as they are manifested and potentially influenced in the therapy relationship."[1]

Through their care and attention for patients, psychoanalytic practitioners facilitate their understanding of how unconscious internal dramas affect their capacities for work, love, and play. These clinicians' work also resembles the work of exorcists. By allowing patients' projections to inhabit them, they *personally* ingest and digest them. Later, and when the timing is right, they reintroduce these projections to patients, allowing for a more mature reintegration. Such exorcism-like processes empower patients to shatter their bonds with internal critics, saboteurs, and other problematic unconscious agents. Clinicians also criticize, in a manner akin to the literary critic's work, problematic self-images, other-images, and repetitive psycho-behavioral patterns.

Why a polemic?

The fast-food nature of global society accelerates at alarming rates, compelling me to explain the intensive, individualistic nature of psychoanalytic psychotherapy before it's too late. These days, even sound mental health—that is, freedom from disabling levels of mental pain, fulfillment in work and social life, an ability to play, and contentment—comes bundled for sale in cellophane-like packages of cognitive behavioral modification combined with psychoactive drugs.[2] The industrialization of medicine unwittingly minimizes, if not erases, our experience of being human. It infuses the public with the promised benefits of algorithmic cures, rendering us little factory parts ready for machining. Compartmentalized, even manual-based mental health interventions, are increasingly promoted—almost exclusively for economic reasons.

These replace deeper probing of the human subject achieved by long-term psychodynamic approaches.

Poisoned by this mechanized view, persons across the globe seek technical interventions to relieve human suffering. For example, iPhone apps offer anxiety-reduction or meditation-proficiency through simple, allegedly effective programs. Insurance company websites recommend exercise, nutritional, and mindfulness programs to enhance health (and, they hope, reduce claims). In contrast, and primarily because of their complexity, the psychodynamic approaches are highly ambiguous. Explaining them is difficult. No computerized application could deliver them. Psychoanalysis is not about medicine, nor is it about education. In fact, the worst thing students of psychotherapy could do to prepare for their careers is to study psychology or psychiatry. These fields promote scientific detachment. Psychoanalytic students would be best served by learning about philosophy, history, drama, or literature—fields offering *real* insights into human subjectivity. These disciplines represent precisely what the depth psychotherapist encounters—the human subject.

In the more than a hundred years psychoanalysis has existed as a profession, the world has witnessed radical paradigm shifts not only in philosophy, science, mathematics, and the arts, but in how we communicate and exchange information, how we participate as makers and consumers in the global marketplace, and how we conceive of ourselves as inhabitants of the Earth. Yet psychoanalysis remains, primarily, imprisoned in the medical model from which it emerged in the late 1800s. The word itself, *psychoanalysis*, suggests a noun-like entity—the psyche—ready for linear, analytic dissection. Similarly, the word *psychotherapy* conjures a mind diseased in some way and subject to a mechanical intervention—the treatment. In the 1970s, Thomas Szasz,[3] a humanistic psychoanalyst well known for his anti-psychiatry views, vehemently criticized these terms. He disagreed with viewing psychoanalysis as a scientific or medical treatment, rendering him pariah-like among his medical colleagues. Our contemporary culture forgets his equally polemical attacks on reductionism and his privileging of the whole human person. The situation calls for a strident counter-attack.

What then shall these practitioners of personal transformation be called? The word *psychotherapist*, used in an interchangeable fashion with psychoanalyst, counselor, doctor, or therapist, reeks of reductionism. It is inaccurate. Consultant sounds too much like a professional offering services to businesses. Helper ranges too broadly. My editor, Andrea, tells me her young daughter, who saw a therapist after losing a grandparent, referred to her as "my special helper friend." Teacher comes close, but psychoanalysts work with only the curriculum provided by their patients. Psychoanalysts and their patients work more like partners, co-participants, further weakening the educational analogy. Facilitators perhaps describes best depth psychotherapists' roles, but it, too, misses the mark. Because we rely on language when we interact with patients, perhaps we psychoanalysts should be identified as applied linguists. We rely upon the types of healing words that Greek playwright Aeschylus' called *iatroi logoi*. On that basis, Szasz suggested depth psychotherapists be called *iatrologicians*. However, even this term falls short. It emphasizes cognition and marginalizes the highly dynamic, interpersonal, and emotional exchange characteristic of psychoanalytic processes. I utilize the term *psychoanalyst*, or the phrase *depth psychotherapist*, until phrases better than "facilitator of transformational encounters"[4] emerge. I intersperse these terms with other, equally accurate phrases like *psychodynamic* or *psychoanalytic psychotherapist*.

For many years, I avoided use of the word *patient*. I believed it implied passivity; I thought it suggested a lack of agency. Many psychotherapists use the word *client*, first popularized by Carl Rogers.[5] However, it, too, sounds business-like. The word *client* also emphasizes cognition, sidelining the emotional nature of change processes. It neglects the suffering that typically causes persons to seek help from psychoanalysts in the first place. I returned to using the word *patient* when I learned it originates from the Latin *patoir*, meaning "to undergo or to suffer."

Who consults depth psychotherapists?

People with a broad array of psychiatric *or* life problems seek help from psychoanalytic practitioners. Some consult them for relief from common psychological symptoms like anxiety, depression, or alcohol or substance abuse. Others seek help with troubled relationships. They find intimacy difficult. Still others feel alienated and seek answers to existential questions—meaning, fulfillment, how to address feeling lost in the world. Echoing their difficulties, patients' expectations differ. Some wish for only a lessening of their pain or an improvement in their relationships. Their interests mimic medical patients who seek treatment for symptoms. They may have no interest in understanding their unconscious minds or elucidating their subjectivities. Some consult depth psychotherapists for emotional support. They want to be more fully seen or heard. But many desire an in-depth exploration of their inner worlds, an uncovering of unconscious motivations, unresolved conflicts, unaddressed conflicts, or previously unknown trauma.

Practitioners treating patients with identifiable mental disorders, like depression or schizophrenia, proceed the way they would with any of their patients. They *frame* the transformative relationship, bring their *presence* to their patients, and engage them in dialogue to address and alter their internal conversations.[6] The psychoanalytic approaches help patients with physical conditions, but in a different way than traditional medical approaches. Patients with schizophrenia or depression are as self-deceptive as the rest of us, and have conflicts, unmet need states, traumas, and other problems with living. Psychoanalysts increase such patients' self-control by developing increased self-knowledge, disrupting self- and other-destructive patterns, and bolstering autonomy. The psychoanalytic approaches have pragmatic benefits as well, often by increasing medication compliance or helping patients face mental illnesses without shame.

Many patients with high blood pressure or diabetes, for example, comply poorly with prescribed treatments. Psychoanalysts help them understand the nature of their conditions, confront the self-destructive nature of non-compliance, and facilitate overall improved self-care. Freeing patients whose internal dramas result in negative self-valuation helps these individuals lead healthier lifestyles overall. Szasz believed *all* medical disorders feature restrictions on personal freedom. Liberating patients from oppressive internal dramas thereby addresses the mental and the physical. Substantial evidence exists to support the contention that psychoanalytic approaches alter brain structure, but I focus here on the *process* of depth psychotherapy rather than on any of its mutative neurological or psychosocial effects.

Psychoanalytic processes unfold in similar ways for persons free of identifiable psychiatric or other medical conditions. Clinicians enable the same transformational relationship for those feeling trapped in difficult life situations—like unsatisfying marriages, degrading work environments, or existential angst. They explore how unconscious dramatic themes prevent these persons from repairing or ending their marriages, from finding fulfilling, satisfying work environments, or from discovering meaning and gratification in their lives. In brief, psychoanalytic psychotherapists address struggles with love, work, or play regardless of patients' reasons for seeking help.

The range of patients just described further validates the problematic nature of the word *therapy*, with its distinct implication of illness. Given the immense power of the medical-industrial complex,[7] the concept of health itself is a potentially controlling ideology. Persons' ingestion of food, consumption of alcohol, and physical exercise has become subject to regulation by institutions. The National Institute of Alcohol Abuse and Alcoholism (NIAA), for example, recently decreed that 1.5 ounces of alcohol intake is acceptable, creating a societal imperative that potentially constricts personal freedom.[8] Some people worry their abstinence from alcohol deprives them of a healthy degree of vasodilation. Others fear their drinking two glasses of red wine per night—an activity common in Europe—renders them alcoholics.

For example, a patient who drinks two glasses of wine per night may wish to explore this habit during a course of depth psychotherapy. His or her physician may have already advised that, according to the NIAA, they are risking their health. In depth psychotherapy, the authority for patients' welfare resides with patients rather than institutions. Psychoanalytic explorations of the meaning of drinking to excess ranges according to patients' perspectives, not society's. Perhaps one patient feels ashamed that others are judging their degree of alcohol intake. Perhaps another fears their drinking signifies a descent into the morass of alcoholism suffered by his or her father. Alternatively, perhaps she enjoys the sensual experience of the wine, studies winemakers, travels to vineyards, and enjoys wine as an aesthetic, recreational experience. Or perhaps, having tried exercise, mild tranquilizers, meditation, or other forms of obtaining relaxation, he determines that alcohol best relieves tension. Ideally, depth psychotherapists facilitate the exploration of these possibilities and more, helping determine the authentic meaning of the drinking for the patient as well as its impact on others around them.

Aaron Schuster[9] uses the protagonist in Blaise Cendars' novel *Moravagine* to bolster his critique of the contemporary concept of health with its metrics, HIPAA rules, and markers. The novel's protagonist, a psychiatrist, considers health an utterly empty concept, representing nothing more than "an ossified and 'normalized' form of sickness," adding that "what convention calls health is, after all, no more than this or that passing aspect of a morbid condition, frozen into an abstraction." Diseases, on the other hand, the psychiatrist remarks, "are a transitory, intermediary, future state of health. It may be that they are health itself."[10] In other words, health is an illusion, an ideology. In truth, we live in various stages of disease, particularly since the body begins degrading after birth. Psychoanalytic psychotherapy evades the health–disease continuum by focusing on patients' experiences in living their lives.

The fragmentation of depth psychotherapy

Rather than seek commonalities and evolve toward cohesion as did other contemporary professions, psychoanalysis has fallen to pieces. A half-century ago, psychoanalyst Leo Rangell decried the splintering of psychoanalysis, noting that the field had already shared "the history of the twentieth century: expansion, diffuse application, use and misuse, explosion, disaster."[11] Paul Stepansky coins the word "fractionation"[12] and, along with Lewis Aron and Karen Starr, worries its lack of coherence threatens its survival as a distinct profession.[13] One of the field's most renowned contemporary theorists, Jay Greenberg, recently proclaimed, "it is very difficult, ultimately, even to say what psychoanalysis really is."[14] The field fragmented, in part, because of the sheer complexity of the human mind, and, in part, because of theorists' narcissism. Psychoanalysts' efforts to understand the determinants of human subjectivity mimics the proverbial blind men studying the elephant. But in this case the elephant is infinite. The ears, eyes, and trunks have been repeatedly observed, identified, and given varied names by different scholars. These psychoanalysts then glorify their particular nomenclature, gather followers into institutes, societies, and editorial boards, and resist efforts to unify even where psychoanalysis becomes the most consistent, namely in actual practice.

A brief overview of the mind's complexity helps explain why psycho-analysis fragmented. We humans tend to turn inward to consciously and unconsciously converse with ourselves. The social philosopher George Herbert Mead observes how humans relate to themselves much as they relate to others, writing: "one is talking to one's self as one would talk to another person."[15] Consciously or unconsciously, people are constantly engaged in internal conversations while, at the same time, conversing with others. We inhabit two parallel worlds, inner and outer. We view the world through the lenses of our internal dramas, which, in turn, run alongside our external ones. Psychoanalysts may be considered professionals who, among their other knowledge bases, have expertise in accessing these dialogues, these internalized schemata, as well as the parallel external, interpersonal ones.

Our inward-turning propensities exist along a continuum. On the conscious end, we harbor thoughts, feelings, and behaviors that we keep to ourselves—negative feelings about friends, envy for colleagues, and the like. These often provide fodder for exploration in psychoanalytic relationships. Moving toward the unconscious, we may harbor dis-sociated mental content, such as disavowed conflicts or deficits. Psy-choanalysts bring these into awareness. The subtle differences between *disavowal* and *denial* provide a useful demarcation. An individual who drinks to excess may know it but ignore it—an example of disavowal. People who drink to excess while oblivious to the frequency or volume may deny their alcohol abuse. The former represents a type of conscious avoidance; the latter is, by definition, unconscious. When your friend, who drinks a bottle of Scotch per night, denies doing so, he or she is *not* lying. He or she does not see it. These examples of disavowal and denial illustrate the conscious-unconscious border. If England represents con-sciousness, and France the unconscious, then the boundary between disavowal and denial lies halfway along the Chunnel running between the two countries.

Further down the continuum are concretized unconscious struc-tures like the id and superego—to use the original Freudian metaphors. Prior psychoanalytic scholars have explored the idea of internaliza-tion, whereby mental content enters the unconscious. They use dif-ferent terms. Ronald Fairbairn's phrase "schizoid background,"[16] for example, or Melanie Klein's "schizoid mechanisms,"[17] name essentially synonymous phenomena. Neville Symington proposes, as I do, that we humans all share such a propensity toward internalization.[18] Again, psychoanalysts work by inviting patients to bring their intrapsychic conversations into the interpersonal realm, creating transformational experiences that, in turn, expand patients' understanding of how these outside-of-conscious-experience themes affect their thoughts, emotions, and behaviors.

Facilitating transformational relationships through framing, presence, and engagement is consistent with any depth psychotherapy school. Essentially, practitioners immersed in Freudian, Kleinian, or Jungian psychoanalysis, or those interested in the more contemporary self-psychological, intersubjective, or relational models, utilize these three modes of intervention. The field of depth psychotherapy could find greater cohesion if its practitioners considered psychoanalytic models as sources of information—symbols, metaphors, signifiers, representations—rather than universal truths. If three millennia of theology and philosophy have failed to identify universals, why would psychoanalysis think it could? I join recent scholars like Jay Greenberg, who likens psychoanalytic theories to "controlling fictions,"[19] or Robert Wallerstein, who believes different psychoanalytic theories offer a "diversity of explanatory metaphors."[20] These scholars utilize the various psychoanalytic theories as useful clinical concepts rather than absolute truths.

The *Lover*, the *Exorcist*, and the *Critic*

Seeking non-scientific and non-medical analogies, I propose three distinct social role analogies for psychoanalysts: *Lover*, *Exorcist*, and *Critic*. Comparing depth psychotherapists to lovers may prove disturbing, even offensive. But this basic truth needs telling: Psychotherapists facilitate intimate, if structured and bounded, interpersonal relationships. Like lovers, mistresses, or paramours, these relationships unfold in private sectors of patients' lives. Since patients pay depth psychotherapists for the services, they behave, in a sense, like sex workers. As I present my three case studies, my description of my work with Gilda specifically reveals the prominent role sexuality can play in psychoanalytic relationships. However, psychoanalytic psychotherapy involves a contractual type of conversation that sexuality, or any overt physical behavior, such as aggression or even massage, disrupts. Nonetheless, because of the crucial importance of empathy, attunement, reception, curiosity, attention, respect, and similarly caring behaviors to psychotherapeutic relationships, I begin with the analogy to lovers.

Once their transformational relationships are properly framed and nurtured by this caring presence, depth psychotherapists receive and contain their patients' projections. They allow patients' internal demons to possess them. They enact roles demanded by these internal scripts, monitoring the media—namely the professional relationship—on which problematic features of patients' internal dramas materialize. By analogy then, psychoanalysts also function as exorcists. As the psychoanalytic relationship becomes shaped by projections from patients' internal dramas, deeper exploration of patients' narratives occurs. I once had a patient accuse me of behaving in a cold and critical fashion toward her; later the same morning, another patient complained of me being too warm. I could not have behaved *that* differently with my two patients. Most likely, projective processes contributed to their differing perceptions. In this manner, depth psychotherapists act like literary critics. They use hermeneutics, the theory and method of interpreting texts, to understand their patients' subjective worlds. These include verbal and nonverbal communication, symbols and signs, and repetitive psychobehavioral themes. Psychoanalyst and historian Peter Loewenberg describes psychoanalysis as "a hermeneutic science of meanings, in which two people together create a secure field for the exploration of latent and least-understood meanings ...," including "fantasies, dreams, sexuality and gender, attachment and losses, interactions (including their dialogic encounter), behaviors, life and death."[21]

When taken together, these analogies to the *Lover*, the *Exorcist*, and the *Critic* most accurately portray what depth psychotherapists *actually do*. I do not mean any derogation in using these metaphors. Instead, I exalt psychoanalytic work, exposing the reality of a profession I have been practicing for more than forty years. I have provided depth psychotherapy for hundreds of people. I have spent thousands of hours intimately involved with them, sometimes four or five sessions per week, sometimes with them lying on the couch while I sit behind them, but more often sitting face-to-face. Perhaps the most overall conclusion I have reached is that an intense interpersonal relationship lies at the heart of psychoanalytic work. And, along with it, all of the frailties, idiosyncrasies, and quirks inherent in all relationships. Emerging from the engagement and safety of that intimate alliance, a live enactment occurs, which, when closely scrutinized and analyzed, alters patients' worlds. It liberates them from destructive, repetitively internalized, and, in parallel, externalized interpersonal dramas. In the quiet confines of my office, I serve as *Lover*, *Exorcist*, and *Critic* day-in and day-out.

Psychoanalysts as *Lovers*

Arguably more than any other profession, prostitution involves the selling of a relationship. Sex workers peddle a particular type of interpersonal engagement, namely a carnal one. Obviously, many sex workers sell themselves out of desperation or financial need; some become prostitutes as a result of sexual slavery, and some sell sex because of trauma. No matter the cause—and likely it is unique to each sex worker—nothing spares him or her from the ultimate fate of becoming an object for another's use, demeaning body and self. Yet sex work most resembles depth psychotherapy. Others have already made the comparison. Cultural theorist Slavoj Žižek writes, "Money—paying the analyst—is necessary in order to keep him out of the patient's pathology." He describes the depth psychotherapist as:

> A kind of "prostitute of the mind," having recourse to money for the same reason some prostitutes like to be paid so that they can have sex without personal involvement, maintaining their distance—here, we encounter the function of money at its purest.[22]

Purest because the exchange evades Marx's idea of surplus value. The psychoanalytic service is clear, the product is custom-made, and it requires clinicians' close attention. Also, it involves talking *about* the service, namely what occurs between the two parties. The relationship between sex workers and customers is more limited. The sex worker sells his or her body for sex, but the relationship ends there. The psychoanalyst, too, sells a relationship, but in a more dynamic, multi-faceted, and bounded fashion. Psychotherapists differ on the degree to which they bring their subjectivities into the healing relationship, but none deny they become personally engaged. An intense, intersubjective relationship lies at the core of the encounter.

In the major professions in our society, such as law, medicine, or accounting, the relationship between professional and consumer is important. But it never forms the core of the work. If you need an attorney, you should seek the one with the best legal skills. Hopefully, you enjoy a pleasant relationship with your lawyer. But what you purchase is a certain knowledge base—writing, rhetoric, argument, or influence. In medicine, the relationship is also important, but, like in law, a set of skills—injections, medications, infusions, radiations—comprise the treatment. Most medical interventions, be it an influenza vaccination, a prescription for hypertension, or a breathing treatment, will be the same regardless of the physician. The accounting analogy follows these closely. The warmth of the accountant enhances tax preparation or auditing processes, but the service lies outside the professional relationship. When purchasing services from psychoanalysts, consumers buy structured, interpersonal relationships intended to transform them personally. Even if different psychoanalysts show similar degrees of empathy for whatever ails you, confront you about self-defeating patterns, or interpret features of your unconscious mind, the experience will certainly be unique. Each depth psychotherapists' personality style, sociocultural background, historicity, and other contextual factors affect the relationship; these same factors affect patients, contributing to the singularity of each psychoanalysis. Each psychoanalyst–patient relationship is inimitable. They cannot be replicated within single sessions or over sets of them. Every encounter is unique.

Furthermore, psychoanalysts lack any distinguishable technique akin to the treatment manuals guiding many behavioral approaches. They *manage* or *facilitate* a transformational relationship. The *being* of the person who facilitates the process, in conjunction with your *being*, overshadows any standardized procedures. If your depth psychotherapist points out similarities between your relationship with your husband and the relationship between your mother and father, he or she will have made an interpretation. Yet—and as those of you who have consulted psychoanalysts will readily agree—the core of the experience is the context, namely the interpersonal relationship in which the interpretation is offered.

Psychoanalysts' interest in, care for, and curiosity in their patients consistently forms the basis for their work. Conservative depth psychotherapists tend to relate to their patients in a formal fashion. They rely on abstinence (avoiding gratifying any of their needs in the process, even, say, their own curiosity about some element of your life) and neutrality (they strive to react evenly to whatever you report, whether a hostile thought or a painful memory). They might strive to *understand* rather than *care* for patients. Nonetheless, and despite allegedly withholding the expression of caring for their patients, they remain closely attuned to them during each session.

Liberal depth psychotherapists use less abstinence or neutrality, may disclose elements of their own lives along the way, and generally rely upon the actual interpersonal relationship as a transformative tool. However, all psychoanalysts use their relationships with patients as the primary means of helping them learn about their unconscious minds. *Transference* refers to the process through which patients project their internal dramas onto their psychoanalytic relationships. Regardless of where psychotherapists lie on this conservative–liberal continuum, they offer transference interpretations. They prevent, or at least minimize, patients' invitations into roles characteristic of their internal dramas. For example, if your internal world features a harsh internal critic, you may unconsciously influence your depth psychotherapist to adopt a critical attitude toward you. You may project the critical part of yourself onto the psychoanalyst. Again, even conservative psychotherapists avoid these types of enactments and, instead, interpret them. Therefore, they, too, use the interpersonal relationship as the crucible of the transformational process. If you walk into a depth psychotherapist's office and perceive the clinician as distant and distracted, walk out. Better yet, run out. Nothing significant can occur in an interpersonal environment lacking an emotional connection. And, thus, the *Lover* forms the first part of the essential social role served by depth psychotherapists.

Psychoanalysts as *Exorcists*

A contemporary interpreter of Freudian psychoanalysis, Jacques Lacan,[23] writes that psychotherapists give their patients three things: language, desire, and being. The language part is simple. Psychotherapists offer any number of verbal interventions, from communicating a sense of understanding (at the most basic level) to communicating a highly complicated interpretation (at the most complex). Lacan's concept of desire is more intricate. Psychoanalysts lend their *own* desire to understand the unconscious mind. For example, a person may be unconsciously invested in viewing their abdominal pain as physical in origin—despite multiple medical evaluations failing to reveal any actual organic basis. Psychoanalysts, in contrast to physicians, bring to the conversation their belief in possibly alternative, unconscious explanations, such as guilt, anger, passive aggression, or loss, manifesting as physical symptoms.

Lacan's final category, namely that psychotherapists also give with their *beings*, helps explain how depth psychotherapists resemble *Exorcists*. Depth psychotherapists take in, and contain—literally psychosomatically—their patients' projections. These features of patients' internal worlds, often painful, and usually immersed in conflict, are projected into others. The logic is simple. People want to rid themselves of pain. Returning to the example of people haunted by excessive self-criticism, they tend to perceive others as critical of them. By unconsciously projecting their internal critic into another person, they lessen their own internal conflict. As a result, and although they may wince in reaction to the criticism from others, or may develop interpersonal conflicts with them, they experience less *internal* discomfort by *externalizing* the conflict. Psychoanalysts become familiar with these projections, understand how to receive them, and explain them. As psychoanalytic boundary expert Glenn Gabbard argues, they "respond rather than react."[24] Often, depth psychotherapists viscerally experience the *being* of the rejecting father, the abandoning mother, or the unappreciative child. Consequently, they feel a wide range of disturbing emotions, from panic to angst, from sadness to unbounded despair, from mourning to melancholia. Psychoanalysts require a high tolerance for pain.[25]

The psychoanalyst Ronald Fairbairn believes practitioners, as Lacan also noted, must engage intensely with their patients to facilitate transformation. He suggests, as I do, that psychoanalysts compete with their patients' devotions to their internal dramas. It's the only family they know. Changing elements of it, even a harsh internal critic, feels like rejection, like becoming an orphan. Like the character of the Jesuit priest played by Jason Miller in the movie *The Exorcist*, psychoanalysts take their patients' experiences into the core of their beings. They regress into the inner world of those who consult them. Regarding these experiences, Fairbairn writes:

> If a True Mass is being celebrated in the chancel, a Black Mass is being celebrated in the crypt. It becomes evident, accordingly, that the psychotherapist is the true successor to the exorcist, and that he is concerned, not only with the "forgiveness of sins," but also with "the casting out of devils."[26]

Using religious imagery, Fairbairn here provides another way of describing how psychoanalysts' *beings* play a central role in their work. He uses the word *exorcist* in literal form. Inventing the phrase *dynamic structures* to describe components of the unconscious mind, Fairbairn hypothesized that patients' "selves" or "egos" exist in close relationship with internal "others" or "objects." An internal critic would be one example of an internal other. Many of you have heard such voices shouting in your own minds, perhaps taking form in thoughts like, "why did I say that to my friend?" or "how could I have behaved so poorly during that job interview?"

In my view, the unconscious mind consists of sets of these internal dramas formed partially by neurobiological propensities, partially by early social learning experiences, and partially by other endless innate and environmental factors. For example, a person with a history of being physically abused may carry within their mind an image of a self-worthy-of-rejection, chronically attacked by a different part of self-identified-with-the-abusive-other. These internal dramatic themes are created during infancy and toddlerhood. Regardless of the hurt they cause, the trends become habitual. Over time, they feel familiar and comfortable. It is not that people enjoy compulsively repeating these patterns; it just feels like home to them. This is why patients, and all human beings, resist change. It is only natural. Why choose orphanhood, even if you find your internal home miserable? Such reasoning forms the best explanation for the well-worn phenomena of resistance.

In the same vein, Fairbairn believes depth psychotherapists must work, arduously, to compete with patients' natural devotion to their internal dramas. The relationship between psychoanalysts and their patients must be intense enough to dislodge such deeply grooved, even unconsciously preferred, internal relationships. Herein also lies the central import of the role of *Lover*. As psychoanalytic processes progress, patients' internal dramas become dislodged, loosened, and disrupted by depth psychotherapists behaving as *Exorcists*. They require a caring reception for whatever follows. I devote an entire chapter to discussing psychoanalytic exorcisms in vivid detail.

Psychoanalysts as *Critics*

Psychoanalysts' use of interpretation forms their main vehicle for their work as *Critic*. They critique, analyze, and offer an understanding of the text of human subjectivity. Psychoanalysts uncover and evaluate various narrative themes guiding persons' images of themselves, others, and their life situations. This critical dimension of depth psychotherapy depends on how deeply patients trust their psychoanalysts, underlining the integrated application of the role of *Lover*. In fact, the roles of *Lover*, *Exorcist*, and *Critic* overlap with one another. Through offering the caring and curiosity characteristic of the *Lover*, psychoanalytic psychotherapists create comfortable sanctuaries and transformational environments, inviting the projections that then possess them in their role as *Exorcists*. As *Exorcists*, they inhabit patients' internal worlds, metabolize them, and reintroduce them to patients. As psychoanalytic relationships intensify, the process of interpretation— involving as much emotional as cognitive understanding—proceeds through practitioners acting as *Critics*. The *Critic* allows for real-time exploration of internal worlds, external relationships, and general lifestyle patterns. Psychoanalysts thereby facilitate exploration of how the internal drama developed, particularly in early relationships with family members and other important figures from childhood; they explore how these recurrent themes present in patients' current relationships. Mimicking the process literary critics use in analyzing texts, practitioners facilitate hermeneutical discussions—analyzing multiple themes and meanings—with their patients. They critically explore myriad manifestations of the unconscious as it presents in verbal material, dreams, slips of the tongue, transference, and elsewhere. Other aspects of patients' lives, such as patterns of relationships, of mood, of interest, of occupational and recreational endeavors, become subjects of study as well.

The inherent artistry of depth psychotherapy

As psychoanalysts gain experience, they develop a singular style, much like accomplished artists find their vision or voice. They learn to improvise. They become skilled at remaining authentic while remaining interpersonally engaged—the theme in Irwin Hoffman's dialectical-constructivist model.[27] By the dialectic, Hoffman refers to the two-part process through which psychoanalysts enact certain dramatic themes while also observing, reflecting, and commenting upon them. By its nature then, depth psychotherapy constitutes an art form. It most resembles performance art.[28] Practitioners undergo extensive training comparable, by analogy, to what art students undergo in their first few years of art education. They study Freud, Carl Jung, Melanie Klein, Fairbairn, Donald Winnicott, Wilfred Bion, and other psychoanalytic theorists. They learn these models of mind; they learn how they foment personal transformation.

However, and strangely, psychoanalysts work in a diametrically opposite fashion from other comparable professionals. Their work radically differs from certain, specific medical specialists, such as surgeons or anesthesiologists. Psychodynamic psychotherapists require the conscious participation of their patients. Their work differs because a specialized, unique kind of interpersonal relationship forms its core. Any professional reliant upon specialized technology automatically differs from the intensely human work practiced by depth psychotherapists. In many ways, psychoanalysts practice the *art* of medicine—but without the medicine. Next, I introduce you to the three vibrant persons who embarked on long courses of psychoanalytic work and entered metaphorical time machines. Their stories will help you understand what depth psychotherapists *actually do*.

Notes

1. Shedler, J. (2010). The efficacy of psychodynamic psychotherapy. *American Psychologist*, 65(2): 98–100.
2. Gnaulati, E. (2017). *Saving Talk Therapy*. Boston, MA: Beacon Press.
3. Szasz, T. (1978). *The Myth of Psychotherapy*, Syracuse, NY: University of Syracuse Press.
4. Karbelnig, A. (2016). The analyst is present: viewing the psychoanalytic process as performance art. *Psychoanalytic Psychology*, 33 (Supplement 1): 153–172. Doi: 10.1037/a0037332.
5. Rogers, C. (1951). *Client-Centered Therapy: Its Current Practice, Implications and Theory*. London: Constable.
6. Karbelnig, A.M. (2022). Chasing infinity: Why clinical psychoanalysis' future lies in pluralism. *International Journal of Psychoanalysis*, 103(1): 5–25.
7. Wohl, S. (1984). *The Medical-Industrial Complex*. New York, NY: Harmony.
8. National Institute on Alcohol Abuse and Alcoholism, No. 16 PH 315, April 1992.
9. Schuster, A. (2016). *The Trouble with Pleasure: Deleuze and Psychoanalysis*. Cambridge, MA: MIT Press.
10. Cendars, B. (2004). *Moravagine*. Alan Brown (Trans.). New York, NY: *New York Review of Books*, pp. 16–17.
11. Rangell, R. (1974). A psychoanalytic perspective leading currently to the syndrome of the compromise of integrity. *The International Journal of Psychoanalysis*, 55: 3–12.
12. Stepansky, P.E. (2009). *Psychoanalysis at the Margins*. New York, NY: Other Press, p. xvii.
13. Aron, L., & Starr, K. (2013). *A Psychotherapy for the People*. New York, NY: Routledge.
14. Greenberg, J.R. (2015). Therapeutic action and the analyst's responsibility. *Journal of the American Psychoanalytic Association*, 63: 15–32. Doi: 10.1177/0003065114561861.
15. Mead, G.H. (1934). *Mind, Self, and Society from the Standpoint of a Social Behaviorist*. C.W. Morris (Ed.). Chicago, IL: University of Chicago Press, p. 141.
16. Fairbairn, W.R.D. (1941). A revised psychopathology of the psychoses and the psychoneuroses. *International Journal of Psychoanalysis*, 22: 250–279.

17. Klein, M. (1946). Notes on some schizoid mechanisms. *International Journal of Psychoanalysis*, 27: 9–110.

18. Symington, N. (2002). *A Pattern of Madness*. London: Karnac.

19. Greenberg, J.R. (2015). Therapeutic action and the analyst's responsibility. *Journal of the American Psychoanalytic Association*, 63: 15–32. Doi: 10.1177/0003065114561861.

20. Wallerstein, R. (2013). Metaphor in psychoanalysis and clinical data. In *Metaphor and Field: Common Ground, Common Language, and the Future of Psychoanalysis*, S. Montana Katz (Ed.). New York, NY: Routledge, pp. 22–38.

21. Loewenberg, P. (2000). Psychoanalysis as a hermeneutic science. In *Whose Freud? The Place of Psychoanalysis in Contemporary Culture*. P. Brooks & A. Woloch (Eds.). New Haven, CT: Yale University Press, pp. 95–115, p. 98.

22. Žižek, S. (2008). *In Defense of Lost Causes*. New York, NY: Verso, p. 24.

23. Lacan, J. (2002). *Ecrits*. B. Fink (Trans.). New York, NY: W.W. Norton & Company.

24. Gabbard, G.O. (2016). *Boundaries and Boundary Violations in Psychoanalysis*. Second Edition. Washington, DC: American Psychiatric Association.

25. Karbelnig, A. (2022). The embodied analyst: the mind-body impact of sustained clinical practice. In *Psychoanalysis and the Mind-Body Problem*. Jon Mills (Ed.) New York, NY: Routledge, p. 349–371.

26. Fairbairn, W.R.D. (1943). The repression and the return of bad objects (with special reference to the "war neuroses"). *British Journal of Medical Psychology*, 19: 327–341.

27. Irwin Hoffman, 1998, *Ritual and Spontaneity in the Psychoanalytic Process: A Dialectical-Constructivist View*. Hillsdale: The Analytic Press.

28. Karbelnig, A.M. (2022). Chasing infinity: Why clinical psychoanalysis' future lies in pluralism. *International Journal of Psychoanalysis*, 103(1): 5–25.

CHAPTER 2

The time travelers

The three patients we follow, Carlos, Gilda, and Penn, metaphorically traveled through time every time we met. Already, and particularly given the fourth dimension, I fear that, without sufficient elaboration, the metaphors of *Lover*, *Exorcist*, and *Critic* lack zest. Therefore, I introduce these three individual human beings, describing their *actual* experiences in depth psychotherapy. Such work viscerally illustrates psychoanalytic processes. As noted in the disclaimer section of the front page, I created these patients using anonymized stories from actual patients, from patients whom I heard about by supervising their clinicians' work with them, from various people I know, and from me. The process of alteration and amalgamation renders these stories essentially fictional. However, and despite their composite origin, the ensuing tales accurately represent what occurs when talking, living, breathing, thinking, emoting, and suffering human beings consult psychoanalysts. Of course, I steadfastly avoided sharing identifying information about any actual patients to protect their privacy and maintain their confidentiality.

Interestingly, my fictional shaping of these case histories takes readers in a Buddhist direction. The Buddha described the self or ego as a delusion. In support of his proclamation, all identities emerge from a complex of biological propensities, early social learning, and cultural influences. The dismantling and reconstructing of self-images comprise much of psychoanalytic processes. The French philosopher Jacques Derrida coined the term *bricolage*[1] to refer to the process of identity formation. We borrow incomplete bits and pieces—some DNA here, some early childhood experiences there, and some influences from culture, history, and everywhere, to form *identities*. Derrida defined *bricolage* as a combination of sources "more or less coherent or ruined." In other words, some identity-contributions combine to create a cohesive sense of self. Others become "ruined" through their splintered, distorted natures. You rarely *choose* what ultimately comprises the narrative you call *self*. Some, like educational achievement, occupational standing, or geographical location, involve personal agency. Other forces sculpt you as life progresses. Some enrich; others traumatize.

Your character—a wonderful word because of its allusion to theater—consists of sets of labels. Using nouns to describe yourself—including your own name—is an exercise in fiction. If you meet a stranger at a party, you may discuss your family status—married, single, with or without children; you may disclose your occupation—teacher, musician, or speech therapist, or; you may share your recreational interests—hiking, bicycle riding, or stamp collecting. These nouns hardly represent your actual living experiences. They function like place markings in a book or addresses on a street—to represent a seemingly fixed aspect of our lives. Less definable are the verbs interspersed between these nouns. These states can only be defined the moment they occur, while anticipating them in the future, or when looking back on them. I *am* excited while touring a National Park. I look forward to it. I remember it with fondness. Novelist Tim O'Brien dramatically illustrates the evolving, and imaginary, nature of our self-concepts when narrating his combat experiences in Vietnam:

> In many cases a true war story cannot be believed. If you believe it, be skeptical. It's a question of credibility. Often the crazy stuff is true and the normal stuff isn't, because the normal stuff is necessary to make you believe the truly incredible craziness.[2]

War stories, like the stories we tell ourselves about who we are, are dynamic. Additionally, portions of the bricolage we call *self* dynamically interact with one another throughout life, and these self-images dance and sway depending upon our interactions with others. Depth psychotherapy processes progress, at least in part, through identifying the nouns, verbs, and narrations binding them. It uncovers the characters enacting their parts in the internal drama of the unconscious mind.[3] Further, it dissects multi-layered subjectivity—the combined hatred and love for self and other, the conflicts between ambition and avoidance, and similar paradoxical trends. Also, and closely related to the idea of freedom, psychoanalysis reverses human self-deception and cultural indoctrination. In his typically polemical style, psychoanalyst Jacques Lacan writes:

> The basic thing about analysis is that people finally realize that they've been talking nonsense at full volume for years.[4]

Most of us have no awareness of the nonsense we speak. And, naturally, the indoctrination, the lies, and the distortions blind us. One cannot see whatever colors tint the lenses through which they view the outside world. Persons' subjective experiences are dynamic, complex, and multi-textured. The frequently extensive length of depth psychotherapy results from how long it takes to understand an individual person. Also, and rather humbling, efforts to comprehend persons' lives inevitably fall short. They might behave in a way surprising even to them; they could encounter a problem that changes them. None of us can ever fully know the *other*.

With these disclaimers in mind, I present the complex, unfolding, and multi-layered bricolages of Carlos, Gilda, and Penn. I venture into their internal lives—their dreams, fears, jealousies, hopes, and more; I describe their external worlds as well, specifically their ways of working, loving, and playing. Any one session delivers but a glimpse of a now-vanished moment, washed away like a sand mandala by an ocean wave. Varying in their degree of distress when contacting me, we worked out the session frequency most suited to their needs. Every session was unique. However, they all involved them becoming "unstuck in time."[5] Our discussions often created distinct surrealistic experiences: Sometimes they perceived *me* as their fathers from three decades earlier; other times I saw *them* as my parental figures.[5] Only after creating

these stories did I realize a commonality in difficulties with father figures in all three cases—a theme almost certainly related to my status as
a cis-gendered male. But, perhaps alternatively, the theme relates to my
status as a father. In any event, here come their stories.

Carlos

I present Carlos first, and with an ironic twist. In my years of writing
and teaching, I have consistently held contempt for psychiatric classification systems. They invite a dangerous reductionism. Patients become
schizophrenics or manic-depressives. Their humanity is marginalized. Michel Foucault identifies such objectification of human beings
in his book *The Birth of the Clinic*.[6] As clinics, hospitals, and similar
institutions evolved, wards were organized by diseases or procedures
rather than persons. You visit your aunt-with-cancer in the oncology
unit. You no longer spend time with your ill auntie. Consider what
is commonly known as *clinical depression*, recognized by the technical phrase *major depression*. If I meet four patients with that diagnosis
in one morning, their presentations can differ markedly. Organizing
them into any one category, in effect, destroys their individualities.
The first patient may experience severe, disabling fatigue due to an inability to sleep. The second may sleep eighteen hours a day. The third may
harbor painful regrets, repeating them endlessly to friends and relatives.
The fourth might be socially withdrawn, only leaving his or her house
once every few months.

The disclaimer being noted, it remains absolutely striking how
closely Carlos' personality style meets the criteria for narcissistic personality disorder (NPD). I do not *see* Carlos, or Gilda, or Penn, for
that matter, as diagnostic entities. Nonetheless, Carlos is astonishingly
self-involved. His bricolage features rigidity, grandiosity in self-image,
selfishness, and lack of empathy. Personality disorder diagnoses refer
to deficits in character itself, in personhood, and in personal style.
Persons whose styles meet the criteria for NPD tend to exaggerate
their self-importance. They overstate achievements and talents. Preoccupied with fantasies of their own success, power, brilliance, or
beauty, they consider themselves superior. Often, they believe only

similarly special people understand them. Others typically view them as arrogant.

A colleague who provided Carlos with four years of twice-weekly psychotherapy referred him to me right after I completed psychoanalytic training. Carlos gained a great deal of self-knowledge through his work with her. He and his prior psychotherapist nonetheless missed significant themes. Carlos continued to experience a sense of tremendous emptiness and loneliness haunting him throughout his life. His rigid but brittle narcissistic shell barely contained such underlying distress. He made no progress in his efforts to reduce his use of alcohol and marijuana. Also, although he felt lonely and isolated, Carlos failed to develop any significant relationships with others.

A specific incident with Carlos' daughter led him to transition to consulting me. She had been accepted into an elite private school which started with kindergarten. Carlos toured the facility. While walking around the school grounds, he felt intense sadness. He was unaware of what triggered the feeling. Within minutes, he began weeping uncontrollably. One of the teachers observed him, assumed care for the child, and allowed Carlos to step outside and compose himself. He described having an "anxiety attack." He realized the warm, accepting school environment—from the lush playgrounds to the high-tech classrooms, from the intelligent, motivated teachers to the welcoming administrators—elicited memories of his completely opposite academic experiences. After finishing the tour, Carlos felt a renewed motivation to "work these issues out." His psychotherapist suggested he undergo a formal psychoanalysis for which she lacked the training. Therefore, she referred him to me.

Shortly after Carlos entered my consulting room, I was struck by his immediate idealization of me. He described his prior therapist as "also a fan"; he referred to my reputation as "off the charts." I greeted him in my usual way, inviting informality by using my first name when introducing myself. He preferred to call me "Dr. Alan." After a few more discomfort-inducing accolades, he explained his relationship with the former psychotherapist. Next, he told me the story of his experience at his daughter's private school. He felt "overwhelmed" by it, adding, "I never cry like that." He found the contrast between the quality of his daughter's school and his often dangerous, poor-quality school experiences as "crushing."

Young, Latino, and working in a business, Carlos looked like he was off to the gym. He was, in fact, on his way to work. He was of average height but substantially overweight, particularly plump at the waist. He still looked good, handsome even, but his puffy bodily appearance detracted from his attractiveness. Although he never graduated high school, Carlos presented as highly intelligent. He enjoyed reading, though he read only biographies of major industrial icons such as J.P. Morgan, Andrew Carnegie, and Joseph Kennedy. He considered them guides for his life. Napoleon fascinated him, and Carlos believed self-interest ultimately killed him off. He hoped his memorizing Napoleon's story might save him from a similar fate.

Carlos described a few other details of his life in our initial session. His grandparents immigrated from Guatemala, but he had no family ties there. He married when he was thirty but never honored the traditional marital contract. He dominated all aspects of the relationship. His wife, Maria, who believed she had married a "great man," submitted to his every whim. He slept in his own room, and he came and went as he pleased. The marital relationship belonged more in the nineteenth century than the twenty-first. The arrangement facilitated Carlos' sexual involvement with other women. An extremely noteworthy fact, Carlos never allowed himself to ejaculate during sexual activities, considering an orgasm as signifying weakness. He ejaculated during intercourse when he (and he alone) decided to have a child with Maria. They had one daughter. Carlos felt disappointed, wishing and even praying for a son. He lived with Maria and their daughter in a guesthouse behind a large house in Torrance, a suburb of Los Angeles.

Despite our divergent backgrounds, Carlos and I related well. He felt connected to me, and I to him. We decided, together and as noted, to proceed with an aggressive, intense psychoanalytic process. We met four, sometimes five, times a week for nearly eighteen months. We both viewed the sets of psychoanalytic encounters as progressing well. Encouraged by the safety I offered him, Carlos shared, to use his words, "secrets I hide from everyone, even me." These included myriad extramarital affairs, his ejaculatory habits, and his deep personal insecurity. His loneliness defied description. He felt orphaned. In a prophetic moment, around two months after we began meeting, Carlos moved his chair closer, knelt in front of me, took my hands in his, and put our interlocking hands onto my legs. He sobbed. Through his tears, he pleaded:

"Will you be the father I never had?"

I remember the moment clearly. I felt awkward, unsure of how to respond.

I looked into Carlos' eyes while pondering my reaction. After a few moments of reflection, I told him, "I will certainly try." My pledge of paternal adoption might seem strange, given my job description and the small age gap between us. But Carlos never enjoyed the benefits of any relationship with a father or even a father-figure. Inverting his intense need to matter to someone, he instead fathered everyone else. He financially supported most of his former parental figures, abusive or not. He called them weekly. As Carlos and I later discovered, these interpersonal patterns resulted from him unconsciously projecting the wounded, yearning part of himself into them. These projections allowed Carlos to retain a position of invulnerability by taking care of the "little boy" in him—but only as he perceived it in others. No one took care of him. Carlos would have resisted any such effort.

Regarding the exorcism theme, Carlos often projected his wounded child-self into me. He strived to protect me as he did other parental figures. He asked questions about my health. He encouraged me to eat properly. Ironically, despite his conscious wish for a father, it remained extremely difficult for Carlos to assume any kind of vulnerable role and, by extension, to *receive* care. Instead, he projected his terrific insecurity into me. I took possession of it. I *felt* insecure like him. Over time, I observed the process, explained it to Carlos, and gently passed the oft-discussed and processed projection back to him. After many months of discussion, we began integrating it back into his own personality. Such a metaphorical exorcism process recurred repeatedly, buttressed by my role as *Lover*. It offered him sanctuary. In my role as *Critic*, I helped him understand, over time, the deeper meaning of this and similarly repetitive patterns.

Carlos' childhood was rife with the type of trauma leading persons to develop narcissistic façades to hide their underlying despair. He grew up in extreme poverty in the South Bay of Los Angeles. His father, who routinely abused his wife and his children, abandoned the family when

Carlos was an infant. Carlos' mother subsequently raised him and his two older half-brothers in garages, in cars, on the street, and in storage units in a predominantly Latino neighborhood. His mother worked two full-time jobs to support the family. His two older half-brothers alternated between neglecting him and beating him. Their mother moved "when the rent came due." As a result, Carlos attended fourteen different elementary schools, disrupting his ability to make friendships or enjoy stability in education. During psychotherapy sessions in which he recalled these isolating, frightening periods, he occasionally wept—an expression of sadness and loss he rarely felt consciously, rarely noticed, and even more rarely, if ever, showed to another.

If an infant finds no support from its mother, it turns to its father. If it finds no comfort there, it turns to itself. The evolution of Carlos' identity strongly validates this well-worn theory of how narcissistic styles evolve. Had he been biologically predisposed, or more severely traumatized, Carlos may well have become psychotic. Or he could have developed a borderline personality disorder (BPD), characterized by instability, disorganization, and fragility. Narcissistic personality styles are, in a sense, an upgrade of a borderline one. Patients with such styles organize themselves around idealized, grandiose self-images. However, inside, they feel fragile, lonely, weak, and unlovable. Carlos had good enough genes, and sufficient positive attachment experiences with his mother, to develop, at least, a narcissistic style. He was, in a sense, lucky. His two brothers became petty criminals. Carlos found a different means of escaping his emotionally and financially impoverished childhood. The primitive kernel of positive self-image gradually grew into unwieldy proportions. As Carlos entered adolescence, he discovered his inherent intelligence. Teachers, employers, and others commented upon it. He quit school in the eighth grade, obtaining employment when he was fourteen. Carlos set out to make a life for himself. He considered formal schooling wasteful. He first worked for a neighborhood diamond dealer who paid him below the minimum wage, and in cash.

Carlos' natural abilities—intelligence, intuition, and courage—led to successive reinforcements of his narcissistic style. He thought he was great, others told him so, and over time such praise bolstered the already-emergent, defensive cover for his deep insecurity. His character armor slowly hardened. When Carlos turned 18, he began working for a national jewelry chain. His superiors quickly promoted him, first to store manager at age twenty and then, at twenty-three, to regional manager. Shortly thereafter, a recruiter offered Carlos a position with a financial services company. The firm had a multi-layered management system that allowed higher-level managers to earn a percentage of those working below them. Carlos remained steadily employed by this firm. He achieved the second highest possible management level nationwide, earning just under $100,000 per month. He worked seven days a week. Like a priest delivering sermons, Carlos spent Sundays giving motivational speeches to his employees. He worked feverishly, as if running from the terror of his early childhood. Ironically, although overtly arrogant in some ways (particularly about his income), he struggled to identify with his own success.

Stuck in the quiet consulting room with me, Carlos found other ways to avoid his underlying emotional pain. The vulnerability inherent in his role as patient gradually became unbearable to him—even though, at times, he regressed with me and revealed the depth of his sadness and sense of loss. After around six months, Carlos began arriving for appointments late. He discussed current events to avoid more intimate topics. Sometimes he began sessions by showing me his sales record, and bragging about his ranking compared to his colleagues. Other times, he asked if we could meet in coffee houses or restaurants. He scoffed when I explained professional boundaries to him.

"Someday you will throw out your ethics book and let me buy you a drink," he proclaimed.

Carlos railed against the ways depth psychotherapists typically frame their professional relationships. His idealization of me persisted. He referred to me as the "best psychoanalyst in California." His narcissistic bubble enfolded our relationship. He was fantastic. So was I. Therefore, he was safe. Despite the intermittent lowering of his defenses, and our both witnessing and being present when displaying real emotional pain, I found our work that "first season" often frustrating. (He used the word "seasons" to describe our work together because it felt to him, in some ways, like an episodic Netflix or Amazon Prime television show.) He often avoided digging into deeper themes. I became more confrontive of his avoiding pain, and of his taking refuge in his "greatness." His regaling me with stories of his success became boring.

At some frustrating point, I retrieved my copy of the *Diagnostic and Statistical Manual of the American Psychiatric Association (DSM-V)*[7] from my bookshelf. I read the nine criteria for NPD to Carlos. He readily agreed, but the intervention failed to break through his grandiosity. If anything, the conversation confirmed how he viewed himself, and his narcissism became further ossified. Next, I explained Melanie Klein's concept of the manic triad[8] to him. She brilliantly identified triumph, contempt, and control as means of avoiding dependency. Here, Carlos again showed total agreement, and seemed proud of these strategies. Ronald Fairbairn,[9] a contemporary of Klein's, considers adulthood as characterized by mature dependency, acknowledging the normalcy of our reliance on others. Rather than call a friend for comfort, a physician for consultation, an attorney for advice, or otherwise "depend" on others, manic defenses are built to (falsely) transcend even basic needs. People with NPD wish for total self-sufficiency. Carlos was always non-defensive in this regard. He boldly proclaimed dependency as weak, wimpy, and lame. Patients' cognitive understanding constitutes only a minor part of transformational processes. Therefore, my sharing information about narcissism-as-diagnosis had no impact. It represented an enactment on my part—a concept soon to be explained. Sometimes intellectual understanding provides an important marker, a kind of cognitive matrix or framework, useful for thinking about their unconscious patterns. But it creates little actual transformation. If it did, self-help books would quickly put us psychoanalysts on the street.

Even though Carlos rarely revealed his vulnerable core to me, and readers can feel my growing frustration, I remained confident about the positive nature of our first period of psychoanalytic work. Over time, his punctuality improved. He again became more emotionally invested, and his trust in me grew. In a shocking and completely unexpected fashion, our work was disrupted when I suddenly became ill. I developed increasingly severe back pain, which my internist diagnosed as a muscle strain. I dutifully complied with the recommended treatment of analgesics, physical therapy, and rest. Nothing helped. The problem worsened. Within a few months, I could barely walk. In retrospect, my failure to more aggressively seek medical assistance ironically demonstrates my own deficits in mature dependency.

Ultimately, I developed flu-like symptoms leading to more tests, followed by a referral to an infectious disease specialist, Kim Rotary, MD. On Friday, June 13 (yes, "Friday the 13th"!), I consulted three different physicians. Kim was my third. She suspected endocarditis—a form of sepsis affecting the heart, and she referred me for a blood culture. The test is an unusual one, requiring technicians to take three samples of blood at 15-minute intervals.

I saw my usual set of patients on Monday, including Carlos, while waiting for my lab results to return. The worst thing I imagined, as I anticipated my follow-up appointment, was a referral to an orthopedic surgeon who might inject corticosteroids into my lower back. The appointment remains seared in my memory. Kim personally summoned me from the waiting room. I limped, slowly and painfully, into her office. Kim motioned me to sit across from her in her personal office. She sat at her desk, frowning.

"You see that you can barely walk now."

"Yes, I know that." I paused and added, "The back problem is worse."

"It's more than that ..." She paused, scratching the back of her neck. She wore her salt-and-pepper hair in a tight bun, donning a long physician's coat, her name embroidered, centered over *Infectious Diseases*, on the right lapel.

"Actually, Alan, you have endocarditis. You need to be hospitalized immediately."

"You must be kidding," I replied. "Can't you just prescribe antibiotics to kill the bacteria?"

"No." Kim paused again. With slight irritation, she said, "You're not hearing me. You need IV antibiotics. You need to go to the hospital *now*."

Endocarditis is an inflammation of the inner lining of the heart caused by infection, in my case a bacterial one. If the bacteria multiply and grow into a stalk—a vegetation—it becomes life-threatening. If it breaks off, you die instantly from a heart attack or stroke. Kim feared a vegetation. Later, I learned the pain in the back was caused by discitis—a bacterial infection of intervertebral disks. Normal bacterial organisms that live in the human mouth somehow leaked into my bloodstream. They journeyed to my back, and they also headed to my heart's aortic valve, eroding it.

Obviously, following Kim's advice, I drove myself to the hospital a few blocks away. A half-hour later, I lay in a hospital bed hooked up to an IV delivering antibiotics to kill the infection and narcotics to deaden the back pain. A fateful coincidence, my appointment with Carlos was scheduled for 1:45 that afternoon. Because Kim's office is close to mine, I anticipated I would easily make my appointment with him. Instead, while driving to the hospital, I made a few brief phone calls—one of them to Carlos. He was probably already in my waiting room by then. He did not pick up. I left him a message telling him I was being hospitalized and promising to contact him as soon as I could. Although I returned to work less than two months later, I did not see Carlos again for six months.

My medical crisis abruptly ended our first season, and the impact on Carlos was profound.

After a two-week immersion in antibiotics and narcotics, a team of thoracic surgeons performed open heart surgery to replace the destroyed aortic valve. I was discharged after twenty days in the hospital. After recovering at home for another few weeks, I began contacting patients. I wondered if any had gone into crisis. Patients already injured by abandonment sometimes experience such a sudden break in the regularity of sessions intolerable—regardless of the reason. Similarly, patients who are uncomfortable with insights gained into themselves, or who otherwise find vulnerability unbearable, might use the break as a reason to discontinue the depth psychotherapy process. As it turns out, only *one* patient quit during that unexpected two-month break: Carlos.

When I returned to my office in late August, I received the following brief voice mail message from him:

"Hey. It's Carlos. I need to take a break." There was no request for a return call or other information. Just those few words.

When we eventually spoke by phone, he told me that once, while I was hospitalized, he called me. Apparently, we talked, though I have no memory of it. According to Carlos, I promised to return his call. I never did. Most of my time in the hospital was a blur. Having developed such an intense relationship with him, I reached out to Carlos several times after I got his voicemail message. I left him two messages, and sent him

one email. I received no reply. After much reflection and, at the suggestion of a colleague, I sent Carlos a handwritten letter in early October.
Still, I heard nothing. Then, in December—a full six months since I had
been hospitalized—he called and left me the following message:

"You helped me a great deal, Alan. But I want you to know that I will
never darken your door again. I will buy you lunch or a drink. I will
take a walk with you. But I will never, ever be your patient again."

I contemplated calling him back immediately. Instead, I waited a
week to see if he would reach out again. I anticipated the sudden display
of my own vulnerability, vis-à-vis the hospitalization, terrified him.
I deliberately created space for him to reflect. A few days later, Carlos
called again, and this time he left me a demanding message:

"I will meet you again under three conditions. You must talk to me,
for free, on the phone. I will only come back once a week. And you must
promise me that I will know immediately if you ever get hospitalized
again."

Notice how each of Carlos' demands placed me, rather than him,
in a vulnerable position—the *sine qua non* of the narcissistic style.
He insisted I provide him with a free service of unknown duration,
relinquish any opinion about session frequency, and offer him personal
access to me, usually reserved for closest relatives and friends. Understanding the sheer terror driving him to such a stance, I called Carlos
back within a few hours. I imagine I passed some kind of a test by agreeing to his first condition. Carlos is not without a conscience (albeit a
compromised one), so he kept the call brief. Of course, I consented to
the decreased frequency of the meetings. Building patients' autonomy
represents one of the few universals across the various psychoanalytic
theories. I encouraged him to wait to discuss the third condition until
we met in person again. Carlos reluctantly agreed.

Carlos and I met for what began our "second season" of work early the
next calendar year. Later in this book, I explain, in detail, the meaning
of him terminating in the way he did. Briefly put, Carlos could not stand
the idea of my being vulnerable—particularly as his own ability to open
up progressed. By the end of that next year, Carlos became increasingly
uncomfortable. Ironically, this time he shared his emotional pain more
openly and frequently. He was less defended. Although I shared some

details of my personal life with Carlos—accommodating his strategy of leveling the playing field and reducing his discomfort—I avoided delving too deeply into my own darkness. Instead, I confronted Carlos with his avoidance maneuvers evident by, fairly frequently, asking me personal questions.

During our second season, external events in Carlos' life changed for the worse. The IRS audited his personal and professional finances. His marriage fell apart. Although Maria remained satisfied with the relationship, Carlos, remarkably, wanted to find more of a "real partner." His confidence in his ability to parent his daughter improved. By the year's end, I could tell that Carlos' tolerance for our sessions was reaching a limit. It seemed like a fair time for him to initiate a break. And yet, he avoided discussing the topic directly. Toward the end of the year, he canceled one appointment late, and then he failed to appear for the next one. When I called him, he claimed his reasons for vanishing were "obvious." Carlos had felt so abandoned at various points in his early life that he simply could no longer tolerate feeling so emotionally vulnerable. At the same time, however, he was incapable of articulating his discomfort. Therefore, he enacted his feelings by disappearing. Rather than encourage an in-person discussion, I facilitated Carlos' taking a second break by phone. I told him I understood his need to stop the regular sessions, and I reminded him that my door would always be open to him.

Carlos has since returned for two more seasons, each one lasting around a year. The intensity of Carlos' emotional injuries, combined with the power of his narcissistic defenses, make psychoanalytic work difficult. His narcissistic style also accounts for why I have thus far enjoyed four seasons of Carlos, and why I anticipate that our work will progress slowly, intermittently, over a period of years. On an intellectual level, Carlos has already come to a clear understanding of how his personality style manifests in his relationship with me and others, like his wife, his employees, his daughter—all *others* in his life. But he clings to it like an addict. He hides his narcissistic retreat, and maintains it, relying on it like a heroin addict on a hit. His style remains, overall, arrogant, superior, and withdrawing. I share much more about Carlos' psychology in subsequent chapters.

Gilda

Gilda reached out to me shortly after the endocarditis misadventure. Her prior psychoanalyst planned to retire, and she wanted to maintain the psychoanalytic work. He referred her to me. Gilda, like Carlos, wanted an immersive psychotherapeutic experience. During our first telephone call, she asked if I could work in several sessions a week with her. I consented. A striking contrast to Carlos' psychological style, Gilda displayed a masochistic one. Her style was less primitive, and yet, like him, her sense of self floated on unstable fault lines. Gilda fully inhabited the deep insecurity that Carlos regularly projected into others. She was plagued by self-doubt. She felt emotionally insecure. She struggled to identify her own desires, instead overly accommodating to the needs of others.

Gilda had met with her prior therapist for ten years on a twice-weekly basis. Knowing of my interest in the humanities, he thought she and I would be a good fit: Gilda had a lifelong interest in history, philosophy, and literature. I lamented not studying these topics earlier in my life. I frantically tried to catch up—listening to lectures on tape, reading the great books, and studying the major philosophers, East and West. One of the few African Americans in the psychoanalytic field, he survived a gun attack by a patient two decades prior. The trauma ultimately caught up to him, and he decided to leave his practice in order to devote time to his wife, children, and grandchildren. Like me, he knew that, all other factors being equal, the personal warmth of the psychoanalyst, as well as his or her personal interests, bode well for establishing positive psychoanalytic relationships.

In her work with him, Gilda addressed the intermittent, severe depression haunting her since her adolescence. She started meeting with him when she was age seventeen. A psychiatrist as well as a psychoanalyst, he prescribed antidepressant medication while providing depth psychotherapy sessions. He assisted her through some difficult periods, particularly her divorce. Her ex-husband tried to wrest from her custody of their one daughter. Gilda's work with him allowed her to tolerate the divorce as well as the many academic and occupational challenges she faced; most significantly, it helped her identify the masochistic themes evident in how she related to her husband and to the men she dated after her divorce. Gilda had found their work extremely helpful. She dreaded his retirement.

Well before Gilda began meeting with me, he worked with her feelings of grief and loss as she faced the end of their psychotherapeutic relationship. Meanwhile, Gilda had become somewhat more self-confident and self-reliant. She had completed high school with honors, and then transitioned, with a merit-based scholarship, to an Ivy-League college. She majored in American history. They held weekly phone sessions while she was away. During holidays and summer breaks, they met in person two times per week. After graduating, Gilda worked odd jobs while she applied for, and was ultimately accepted into, a doctoral program in history. After obtaining her doctorate, she struggled to find a tenure-track university faculty position. The jobs were scarce. Gilda ultimately accepted a research position for a think-tank affiliated with the US Defense Department. Her prior psychoanalyst announced his intention to retire shortly after Gilda began working there. She had just turned twenty-eight.

Following Gilda's lead, our sessions initially focused on working through her reactions to her previous psychotherapist's retirement. We also met two times a week. Despite her having discussed the retirement with him, she still felt angry at, and abandoned by, him. She feared her psychological difficulties had overwhelmed him, contributing to, if not actually causing, his retirement. She doubted I could be as helpful to her as he had been. As our work progressed, I suggested increasing session frequency to four times per week because Gilda remained, despite her prior work with my colleague, significantly depressed. Also, even though the pattern had lessened in intensity, Gilda still related to others in her life in a masochistic manner. She behaved in an excessively sacrificial way with her daughter, with men she dated, and with friends. I believed that the increased session frequency would bring her emotions, as well as these behavioral patterns, into clearer view. She consented.

Whereas I enjoyed working with Carlos, and liked him, I found the work with Gilda much more gratifying. Gilda brought her vulnerability to the fore without any overt defensiveness. Also, I felt intensely physically attracted to her. Tall, of Greek origin, and extremely articulate, she was a statuesque beauty, taller than me at 5 foot 10 inches. I felt entranced by her wavy brown hair and clear brown eyes. More than purely sexual attraction, Gilda's keen intellect also captivated me. She seemed to have read everything in literature, philosophy, and political science, not to mention history. My attraction only increased as she shared stories of how much she had enjoyed married life—including how easily she regressed into loving sexual encounters with uninhibited pleasure. She genuinely enjoyed the roles of wife, homemaker, and mother, and managed them while actively pursuing her intellectual interests. It was a rare and unusual combination.

Whereas Gilda's prior psychoanalyst had been twenty-five years her senior, I was ten years older than her. Our age difference, particularly compared to her previous therapist, seemed to facilitate my fantasies of romantic engagement. Gilda denied any romantic attraction toward her prior analyst. She viewed him as a paternal, or even grandfatherly, figure. In contrast, she told me she found me "good-looking and kind." Naturally, I kept my feelings for her to myself. Much more on this later, but psychoanalytic relationships require what psychoanalyst Lewis Aron calls "mutual but asymmetrical" intimacy.[10] Therefore, psychotherapists and their patients might often develop intimate feelings for one another, but practitioners rarely share *these* feelings. When and if they do, their self-disclosures ideally move the psychoanalytic process forward in some way. With Gilda, and perhaps due to the degree of my attraction, I brought extra care to boundary maintenance. I listened to her occasional descriptions of attraction to me, or fantasies about my private life. I never responded in turn. Also, I sensed a certain vulnerability in her. I framed our professional relationship in the usual fashion, beginning and ending sessions on time, maintaining a regular meeting schedule, and billing her for my services at the end of every month.

After a few months, our discussions transitioned away from her last psychotherapist to exploring the deeper unconscious themes troubling her since adolescence. Gilda endured severe sexual and emotional abuse during her childhood. Her highly narcissistic parents—both physicians specializing in internal medicine—divorced when Gilda was twelve. Gilda believed that her father disliked her and competed with her.

Even when she was a young girl, he repeatedly told her she was "dumb" and "ugly." To this day, her father shows little interest in her. When she was age nine, Gilda discovered her father engaging in a homosexual extra-marital affair. It involved one of her parent's medical partners, and Gilda knew him. She saw him at the occasional social gatherings at her house.

As if this knowledge were not sufficiently traumatic, the secret romantic partner, a bisexual man, molested Gilda on two occasions. He fondled her when she was five; he sexually assaulted her when she was thirteen. Gilda fended off the latter attack, which occurred when he arrived early for a business meeting at her house. Her parents were still in their professional offices. When they arrived home, Gilda's mother criticized her for appearing unkempt. Her dress was wrinkled and askew because of her struggle with the man. Gilda said nothing. In fact, she never disclosed the abuse to either of her parents. Overall, her mother seemed "lost in her own world," incapable of countering the abuse Gilda received at the hands of her father or his lover. By the time she entered elementary school, Gilda had already oriented herself to satisfy the needs of others. She was unconsciously repeating a relational theme with roots in her early relationship with her father, with his partner who abused her, and with her mother. Gilda already showed, even at that tender age, little capacity for identifying her own needs.

The internal drama related to Gilda's childhood experiences entered the psychoanalytic field during the first few months of our work together. Particularly poignant was our discussion of how her negative sense of self influenced our work. Gilda feared I would abruptly end the treatment, reduce its frequency (out of my presumed resentment because I lowered my fee to facilitate her affording more frequent meetings), or become ill (which I did at one point that first year, causing a one-week disruption in our sessions). Typical in facilitating the depth psychotherapy process, I offered Gilda mostly my role as *Lover* during our initial months of work. I listened carefully. I invited Gilda to wander in her expression of thoughts, memories, and dreams. Later, the *Exorcist* entered our work. I had periods in which I became identified with Gilda's hated-self. During these times, she subjected me to the type of brutal attacks that characterized her internal relationship with herself. She accused me of caring insufficiently. She raged at what she perceived was my objectification of her. (I recall worrying about these accusations because, of course, Gilda sensed my attraction despite my best efforts to hide it.) On occasion, and paradoxically, she expressed fury at the limits of our professional relationship. During these periods of anger—particularly if there had been no real breach like my being late or distracted—I interpreted Gilda's attacks as mimicking her highly critical, shaming internal ones. In attacking me, she was really assaulting herself.

In retrospect, I believe Gilda's intermittent fury at me related both to her unconscious dramatic themes and to residual feelings surrounding her last therapist's retirement. I absorbed Gilda's psychological assaults on me—much like I had with Carlos. Unlike others in her life, I did not react. I brought them to her attention. I commented on them. Later, when a clear pattern emerged, I tentatively offered an interpretation, a hypothesis if you will, of the projective dynamic. Gilda, brilliant as ever, clearly saw the themes once presented. She understood how, in dramatic terms, she had projected her hated-self into me. Through patient discussion, repeatedly, I metaphorically handed the projection back to her. Also, we worked our way through any of the anger I actually elicited, such as taking her into sessions late. The acute episodes of anger diminished by the end of our first year of work. Meanwhile, Gilda had developed an increasingly strong dependence on me.

Enacting the role of the *Critic*, I often interpreted the masochistic features of Gilda's personality style as it manifested in our relationship and elsewhere. Our frequent discussions of the erotic elements of the transference, while consistently maintaining the professional *frame*, caused them to lessen in intensity. Gilda came to understand that at least a component of her attraction to me represented a repetitive pattern formed from the primitive ways she had attempted to get her father's attention. Through such discussions, these and other features of Gilda's internal drama gradually changed. Her inner persecutors became less punitive; her sense of her own value increased. She began to understand the concept of reciprocity in interpersonal relationships.

As I explain in greater depth later, Gilda's generally masochistic style inevitably entered our relationship. Interestingly, the self-defeating theme emerged more noticeably after her anger at me diminished. If she were even a few minutes late, she would apologize excessively.

If I misunderstood a word, or misheard her, *she* apologized. More nuanced than the typical exorcisms characteristic of depth psychotherapy processes, these behavioral patterns elicited in me a sense of hyper-responsibility, of caution. I feared hurting her feelings. Why? Because, in contrast to the times I took on the role of her hated-self, she, at other times, projected her internal critic into me. She expected me to rail against her at any time. Her propensity to apologize defended her against such expected criticism. I took both *dark spirits* from her, processed them, and returned them to her in less inflamed conditions. When I presented, and we discussed, the various themes related to her projection, I was assuming the role of *Critic*. She gained immense insight into numerous self-defeating patterns—like her excessive apologies—as they manifested in her life with me and in her outside life.

Gilda's interpersonal relationships also gradually evolved in a positive fashion. Her romantic life had featured a series of failed relationships, usually casting her in the role of the "supporter" to highly egocentric men. Most of these failed. At the time that Gilda entered the analysis, she was around a year into one of these sadomasochistic relationships. Shortly thereafter, Gilda ended the relationship—that being the first ending of a romantic relationship initiated by *her*. She learned to evaluate the men interested in her with a greater capacity for sensing *their* capacity to behave in an interpersonally mature fashion.

Unfortunately, and in the midst of these positive changes, Gilda sustained an injury that immediately dominated our psychoanalytic discussions. Gilda attended a holiday party near the research facility where she worked. After it, a group of teenagers attacked her, robbed her, and threw her against a brick wall. She sustained injuries to her cervical spine severe enough to require emergency repair of a ruptured intervertebral disc. The surgeon placed her on an extended medical leave of absence. In the months following the assault, Gilda felt even more traumatized because neither her supervisor nor her colleagues contacted her. One female colleague, whom she considered a friend, reached out— but only once. No one else expressed concern for her. The firm's human resource department only contacted her weeks after she was released from the hospital, and this was to discuss the status of paying her disability and health benefits.

Gilda's relationship with me abruptly changed after the attack. She seemed defenseless. She openly described, sometimes in excruciating detail, the depth of her terror. She feared the attack would recur. Her sleep was disturbed by nightmares, causing her to feel exhausted during the day. Gilda displayed classic symptoms of post-traumatic stress disorder (PTSD), including recurrent recollections of the assault, chronic anxiety with intermittent panic attacks, and dissociative episodes. The latter states, also known as psychogenic fugues, were particularly alarming. Estranged from her ex-husband, Gilda reared her daughter without support from him or other family members. During these dissociative episodes, Gilda wandered away from her apartment, often in the middle of the night, prompting her daughter to call the police and me. Because of the potential for danger, I referred Gilda to a psychopharmacologist who prescribed minor tranquilizers for the acute anxiety and sedatives for sleep.

Also, after the attack, and because of these fugue episodes, I began meeting with Gilda on a six-day-a-week basis—a first for me in my career. Those sessions, in conjunction with the change in her medication regimen, caused the psychogenic fugue states to lessen in intensity. They occurred less frequently; they lasted for briefer periods. Meanwhile, I felt compelled to rescue her after she was attacked. I obsessively worried about her. I, too, had trouble sleeping, fearing Gilda would be hurt, raped, or killed, during one of the fugue episodes.

Gilda's acutely traumatized state stimulated the intrapsychic assaults characteristic of her internal drama. She felt ashamed about how she had reacted to the attack, believing she *overreacted*. She thought she had contributed to the assault in some way. Had she left the party too late? Had she failed to park her car in a well-lit area? Her intense self-criticism aggravated the PTSD. Also, her reactions evoked features of my own internal drama, leaving me increasingly desperate to rescue her. Interestingly, though, the severity of her distress caused my attraction to her to transition into more of a paternal, protective one.

The crisis period dominated our third year of working together, during which I felt fully absorbed in my clinical role. Gilda clearly identified with the patient role. Maintaining boundaries became easier—even though we met almost daily. As I will discuss in later chapters, I assumed mostly the role of the *Lover*, the caring other, while the PTSD was acute. No real exorcisms occurred. Even my role as *Critic* became rare. I mostly listened to Gilda shriek and cry her way through that awful period. She became even more intensely dependent on me. After the long period of recovery passed, I began crossing some professional boundaries that deserve much greater attention. I dive deeply into that period later in this book. In brief, our relationship deteriorated, improved, and then ended.

Penn

Unlike Carlos and Gilda, Penn's psychological discomfort never met the criteria for any diagnosable mental disorder. Our work together allows you to gain an understanding of the many ways depth psychotherapy concerns itself with much more than symptom reduction. Of course, my conversations with Carlos and Gilda strayed widely. They covered varied aspects of their lives. But the first two patients had clear and overt symptoms, often severe ones. Penn struggles with anxiety, sometimes mightily. One of my longest intermittent patients—he's been consulting me for nearly thirty years now—Penn has mostly used the meetings to confront problematic themes in his life, particularly his excessively harsh attitude toward himself and his propensity to use devotion to work and productivity like an alcoholic uses hard liquor.

A thin, almost gaunt, Caucasian man who stands some 6 foot 6 inches, Penn appeared tired, worn out by the anxiety that, he said, was at the core of his being during his childhood and adolescence. If I were completing an insurance form, I would denote a diagnosis like generalized anxiety disorder (GAD), or another type of anxiety-related condition, with a clear conscience. But for the most part, Penn's anxiety, and his life difficulties, failed to meet the criteria for any psychiatric classification system. He suffered more from existential issues than psychological ones. Over the course of our work together, his terrors lost their valence, and Penn became entwined in coping with other life problems.

Penn first sought me out because of a "nervous breakdown"—his phrase—that occurred during his senior year of pre-med studies at UC San Diego. He planned to attend the Keck School of Medicine at the

University of Southern California that fall. However, because of the intensity of his distress, he asked for, and received, a one-year deferment. At the start of his last semester, Penn remembers feeling worried about his capacity for sleep, imagining "the disaster" that would occur if he had ongoing insomnia. One night, he thought about that idea so intensely that he only slept an hour or two. He felt acutely anxious the next day. The following night, Penn was unable to sleep at all. He panicked. He imagined failing, the university precluding him from graduation, and the medical school refusing him entry.

As the months passed, Penn grew increasingly convinced that panic, insomnia, and the resulting fatigue would prevent him from achieving his wish for a career in medicine. The frightening thought became an obsession. Penn consulted a cognitive behavioral psychologist at the UC San Diego counseling center. She taught him relaxation exercises to reduce his anxiety and to improve his sleep. She also referred him to a psychiatrist who prescribed a mild tranquilizing agent. Penn was so fearful of becoming dependent on the substance that he used it once or twice, and he then flushed the rest of the pills down the toilet. He never consulted the psychiatrist again. The calming exercises and the medication allowed him to sleep better. They reduced his anxiety. But he continued to feel "haunted" by thoughts of failure.

Already, Penn's story exemplifies the oppressive nature of psychiatric classification systems. In retrospect, Penn likely met the criteria for a mental disorder when I first met him—but only if significant contextual factors are ignored. He never played; he never had fun. Penn was the pre-med student of pre-med students: He studied before breakfast, ate alone, attended his classes punctually, and studied during all breaks, even while eating lunch and dinner. After dinner, he followed the same routine until midnight each night. The next day— rinse and repeat. His few friendships were not particularly intimate; they consisted of "study partners." He called his parents once a week, not feeling particularly close with any of his family members or other relatives. Penn's world consisted of studying and achieving. Nothing else mattered. His problem, on the deepest level, was self-deprivation to the extreme. No wonder he felt terror. Noteworthy for more reflections on diagnostic classification systems, Penn *always* remained highly functional during his emotionally difficult periods. Despite his terror of failure, he never *actually* failed. He performed extremely well in his classes. He completed his studies at UC San Diego, ranking near the top of his class with a 4.0 GPA. Although Penn had always been functional, he often felt miserable. The turmoil he can experience—the obsessive ruminations, the conviction of his inadequacy, and his emotional insecurity—can assume breathtaking proportions.

During those first few years of working together, Penn and I immersed ourselves in discussing the severity of his single-focus life. Penn loosened up a bit. He worked in a lab in Barcelona the summer before he started medical school. We took a break from sessions while he was gone, and then we met again for a few months before he left for school. Meanwhile, one glitch existed in his work-addicted soul, and that concerned his relationships with women.

Penn had a steady romantic relationship with one woman, Gillian, whom he met during his junior year of high school. She attended UC Santa Cruz. They attempted to maintain a long-distance relationship during their undergraduate years, but they grew apart while Penn had his year off. Penn ended the relationship just before he left for Barcelona. Whereas we had focused initially on his blinding devotion to his studies, our discussions abruptly turned to the break-up, which elicited its own dark despair. It also lit up the insomnia problem. Penn felt concerned with how dependent he could become on women—a topic we pursued, in detail, in later periods of our work. The summer in Spain was "an entirely miserable experience." He missed Gillian despite him ending the relationship. He suffered deep bouts of loneliness and alienation. Even months later, he felt "gun-shy" about dating.

Penn's childhood experiences shed light on the life patterns that led him to consult me in the first place. Much like Carlos' and Gilda's early childhood experiences, Penn was severely neglected during his infancy. His mother, a chronically angry, self-absorbed woman, felt angered at her homemaking role. She had five children. Penn was her third child, and her only son. She was overwhelmed by her two eldest children, leaving her "always angry" by the time Penn was born. She projected her disappointment at how her own father treated her and her sisters onto him. She disliked men. Penn's earliest memories of her are of her angrily cleaning the house, washing clothes, or doing dishes. He felt terrified of her. When he was in the third grade, she met him at the front gate when he had friends with him. In front of them, she proclaimed that if he insisted on allowing them into the house, she would not provide milk, cookies, or attention. They would be on their own. That was the last time Penn invited friends over.

Penn's father, a professor of cultural anthropology at a small liberal arts university, behaved in a tender and loving fashion toward him. He achieved tenure at around the time Penn was born. However, he spent much of his time at the university, teaching, serving on committees, and writing. He was much more present in Penn's life than Carlos' or Gilda's fathers; he was more present than Penn's own mother. Penn remembers waiting in the family room next to the attached garage every evening, listening for the sound of the garage opening. It signaled the arrival of comfort.

When Penn entered early adolescence and showed some mild rebellious behaviors, his mother was completely intolerant. She grounded him; she refused to prepare meals for him. Over the next year, their relationship turned still more contentious. His earlier stance of, essentially, cowering in fear around her, reversed itself. He was constantly enraged with her, and she responded with still more verbal abuse. She repeatedly slapped him across the face. Child abuse laws had not yet been enacted, but teachers and students commented on the red welts on his face and neck. Seeking more distance from him, Penn's mother insisted he spend his time during summers and school breaks with his father at the university. His father complied. He assigned Penn a variety of clerical tasks, paying him $1 an hour. Penn enjoyed the time away. It offered him a welcome refuge from his mother. It allowed some passive expression of anger at her: *He* had plenty of time with his father but his mother did not.

On the way to his father's office one day, when Penn was fourteen, he asked his father why he had married his mother. His father was silent. But, after that point, a distinct change occurred in their relationship. His father hid behind his mother, a phenomenon Penn and I came to understand as a "double abandonment." The loving reception Penn expected from his father waned. They drove to the office in silence; at home, Penn's father rarely interacted with him. Penn has only hazy memories of the rest of his childhood, save feeling lonely and isolated. Penn has since struggled with ambivalent feelings toward his father. On the one hand, his father literally saved him emotionally and, quite possibly, physically. On the other hand, Penn viewed his childhood as essentially ending when his father withdrew from him.

In the years after that fateful interaction in the car, Penn's father helped him obtain regular, part-time work at the university. He worked there for the rest of his adolescence. He excelled academically, using his studies and subsequent occupational pursuits as ways to avoid his mother. These activities bolstered his self-esteem and self-confidence. Over time, however, Penn excessively sought refuge in these activities. He failed to develop an ability to become intimate with others, to play or recreate in any fashion, or to otherwise develop more flexible ways of identifying his wishes and satisfying them. He became a workaholic.

Even this brief overview of Penn's childhood explains the evolution of the life difficulties leading Penn to begin depth psychotherapy with me those many years ago. Of course, he would feel terror at the prospect of insomnia or of any problem diverting his tunnel-vision-like life focus. He had no other way to cope with the feelings of terror that lay beneath his only way of feeling worthy. The intense emotional bond he enjoyed with Gillian offered him the maternal attention for which he yearned so intensely. Losing Gillian retraumatized him—even though it was Penn who let her go. He feared their love would adversely affect his goals. He responded with even greater devotion to work and productivity, increasing his emotional deprivation, leading to more terror and insomnia, and so on endlessly.

Just recently, Penn returned for another set of sessions with me. Now forty-eight, he describes a sense of emotional disconnect from his wife and two sons. The children are in their twenties and live in different states. They are financially independent. One works a part-time job while attending a four-year law school; the other manages three Starbucks stores while attending a company-sponsored MBA program. A successful orthopedist, Penn developed a specialized procedure for performing hip replacements early in his career. He became well known, financially successful, and flooded with more patients than he could treat.

Although periods of improvement have occurred along our long journey together, he has recently regressed back into a life of work, work, and more work. He told me:

"I have checked every box in terms of life achievement, and yet I'm empty."

Also, he reports feeling bored. In our last session, he said with a flat voice:

"My work amounts to little less than a mechanic for human bodies."

For a few minutes after he uttered these statements, I felt hopeless. I kept the emotion to myself. Later, I, of course, worked through the rest of Penn's feelings with him, got out my appointment book, and together we set up a schedule for weekly appointments. We shall have another stab at this! As with Carlos and Gilda, I provide multiple examples of how I worked as a *Lover*, *Exorcist*, and *Critic* with Penn later on. My role as *Lover* was both enhanced and complicated by the many ways I personally identified with Penn. I had a similar childhood experience, and similar compulsive leanings. As a result, it was easy for me to offer empathy and support. I got the story; I understood him. Sometimes I grew impatient, though, with the stubborn rigidity of his extreme, almost religious, devotion to accomplishment. I feel it as I write these words now, the frustration, the struggle to help him find the acceleration velocity to emerge from the gravitational pull that keeps him imprisoned in this life pattern.

Over the years, I have served as *Exorcist* with Penn in several distinct ways: I received projections of harshly critical parts of him, of terrifically wounded parts of him, and of dark feelings of isolation and loneliness. Typical of metaphorical exorcist processes, I contained these emotional states, detoxified them, and, over time, gently and gradually reintroduced them back into him. The process enhances his personal awareness and power. As occurs in work with all patients, the *Critic* typically overlaps with the *Exorcist*. It certainly did with Penn. Each exorcism was followed by discussions of how and why these occurred. Additionally, Penn and I reviewed many problematic themes running through his life. Thomas Szasz once quipped that patients come to therapy with solutions rather than problems.[11] The solutions *become* the problems. Penn clearly exemplifies Szasz' point: His excessive devotion to achievement creates feelings of self-worth, but at the price of isolation and exhaustion.

These introductions to Carlos, Gilda, and Penn provide you with glimpses of what typical patients of depth psychotherapy are like, and of what psychoanalytic encounters look like. But, so far, you've seen only a few scenes, a few images. The previews now complete, I next offer more background—specifically the complex philosophical foundations that lie beneath the psychoanalytic project.

Notes

1. Derrida, J. (2001). Structure, sign, and play in the discourse of the human sciences. *Writing and Difference.* Alan Bass (Trans.). London: Routledge, pp. 278–294.
2. O'Brien, T. (1990). *The Things They Carried.* New York, NY: Broadway Books.
3. Karbelnig, A. (2017). The geometry of intimacy: love triangles and couples therapy. *Psychoanalytic Psychology,* 35(1): 70–82.
4. Lacan, J. (2002). *My Teaching.* New York, NY: Verso, p. 71.
5. Faulkner, W. (1951). *Requiem for a Nun.* New York, NY: Random House, p. 85.
6. Foucault, F. (1973). *The Birth of the Clinic: An Archeology of Medical Perception.* Alan Sheridan Smith (Trans.). New York, NY: Vintage Books.
7. The American Psychiatric Association (2019). *Diagnostic and Statistical Manual 5 (DSM-V).* Washington, DC: The American Psychiatric Association.
8. Klein, M. (1946). Notes on some schizoid mechanisms. *International Journal of Psychoanalysis,* 27: 99–110.
9. Fairbairn, W.R.D. (1952). *Psychoanalytic Studies of the Personality.* London: Routledge.
10. Aron, L. (1996). *A Meeting of Minds: Mutuality in Psychoanalysis.* London: The Analytic Press, p. 43.
11. Szasz, T. (1988). *The Myth of Psychotherapy.* Syracuse, NY: Syracuse University Press.

CHAPTER 3

Psychoanalysis' philosophical and historical context

An infinite number of complicated, dynamic forces create human subjectivity. Much will remain forever mysterious. Nonetheless, scholars throughout history have grappled with it. And they have provided many of the underpinnings on which the profession of depth psychotherapy rests. Western thought only liberated itself from religious influences a few centuries ago. From the time Christianity dominated Rome in the 4th century until the Enlightenment began in the mid-17th century, myriad fields of study were dominated by the Church. Arguably "fields of study" is incorrect. All disciplines existed under theology. For the first time in nearly two millennia, scientific realms of study became separated from religion—a radical evolution in the history of ideas. Shortly thereafter, physicists distinguished themselves from chemists who, in turn, studied different phenomena than biologists, botanists, and astronomers. Anthropologists could study civilizations, geologists the earth, and meteorologists the weather.

With the Enlightenment, a schism in thinking, a duality, emerged, and it retains an international monopoly. On the one hand, knowledge in the various scientific disciplines expands exponentially. On the other, the experience of being human remains ever more marginalized.

Sciences' eclipsing of the centuries-long interest in human beings—blossoming in history, philosophy, and politics—progressed into what philosopher Ken Wilber terms the "flatland."[1] Humanism, an interest in human experience, freedom, and personal agency, became replaced by the scientism and empiricism.

In confirmation, Foucault[2] believes, technology's rise parallels the declining interest in subjectivity. Using medicine as an example, he describes how the physician's "gaze" turned away from patients' experiences. Whereas physicians had, for generations, listened to them, hearing stories of their lives, they began objectifying them. Beginning with the stethoscope, and leading rapidly to other investigative modes, physicians peered *into* human bodies. Their focus further marginalized their patients' subjective experiences. Patients became designated by disease types, i.e., the orthopedic floor or the cancer unit, becoming increasingly separated from their personhoods.

Such a post-Enlightenment manner of viewing matter, things, or ideas as linear, as structured into neatly organized matrixes, partially reversed itself beginning in the early twentieth century. Some identify the sinking of the Titanic in April 1912 as the start of science's decline. Considered the paragon of engineering, the unsinkable vessel sank on its maiden voyage. The kingdom of science came under greater scrutiny as the horrors of the Holocaust entered global consciousness a few decades later. The mass extermination of specific religious and ethnic groups grudgingly brought attention back to human persons. How could one of the most culturally sophisticated and scientifically advanced nations come under the spell of a mass-murdering dictator?

Meanwhile, scientific discoveries during each passing decade disrupted the previously ordered sensibility of the physical world. Albert Einstein's theory of relativity[3] revealed a continuum of space and time, and an equivalence of matter and energy. Werner Heisenberg's uncertainty principle[4] inserted human subjectivity into the heart of science: Measurement varied according to the point of view of the observer. And Kurt Godel's theorem of incompleteness[5] eroded the alleged perfection of mathematics. Constructing a complete map of the universe must include the process of the mapmaker making the map, he thought. Paralleling these modernism-destroying events, developments in linguistics and philosophy rendered scientific discourse contextual.

Ludwig Wittgenstein,[6] for example, considered the sciences as simply a variety of language game; Thomas Kuhn[7] showed how personal, human fallibilities contributed to paradigmatic shifts. Postmodern philosophers such as Jacques Derrida[8] and Hans-Georg Gadamer[9] considered post-Enlightenment, scientific categorizations entirely context-based and relativistic. The previously, albeit imaginary, solid ground beneath the scientists trembled.

Scholars of disparate fields of study soon discovered that their disciplines, too, lacked definitive starting or ending points. Physics cannot definitively declare it has found the smallest particle; astronomers see no end to the universe. No comprehensive organizing system, whether looking at things small or large, exists. Even if believing the Big Bang theory, you are left with the daunting question of what happened *before* it. The incomplete, fragmented nature of contemporary knowledge renders the ultimate underpinnings of any field of study mysterious. Therefore, the foundation of an endeavor to seek philosophical foundations for psychoanalysis necessarily rests on a precarious footing.

Illustrating my point, consider your experience in this moment—reading this collection of letters organized into words, words into sentences, and sentences into paragraphs. These entities emerge from irreducibly complex causative factors. Starting from the ground on which you lie, sit, or stand, your geography and country influence your experience. Broader cultural factors, like your level of education and your socioeconomic status, influence your perception. Your biology, dependent as it is on the air you breathe, the fluids you drink, and the foods you ingest, shapes your experience as well. Your early childhood environment, traumatic or supportive, further molds you. These and other factors exist in dynamic interaction with one another, changing over time, delivering to you the enigmatic, unique human experience of this moment. We need not fear it. Perhaps we should feel awe at it. We are spinning, emerging enigmas, each of us unique and ever-changing. Darwin's final sentence when describing biological diversity in his famous *Origin of the Species*,[10] "the grandeur of it all," expresses the inscrutability of it. How do we build organizational structures from such swirling dynamism?

I begin by considering what occurs during any depth psychotherapy session. After properly framing the professional relationship, practitioners receive, with as much openness as they can, the experience of the human subject before them. The role of *Lover* provides as much reception, safety, and openness as possible. Their work as *Exorcists* and *Critics* facilitates additional self-exploration. Along the way, these overlapping roles allow psychoanalysts' patients to resolve conflicts, address deficits, attend to trauma, and grow beyond developmental obstacles. Applying Jacques Derrida's idea that we humans create and play with our *structures of experience*, depth psychotherapy progresses through identifying, uncovering, disrupting, reorganizing, altering, and repairing these structures. Meanwhile, and layered upon the ultimate foundational mystery, four basic philosophies, essentially organizing systems, underly psychoanalysts' work. These systems consist of phenomenology, perspectivism, holism, and existentialism. Obviously not providing complete stability, they nonetheless construct an undergirding for understanding psychoanalysis. Each concerns patients' subjectivities. After introducing the philosophies, I utilize my first few encounters with Carlos, Gilda, and Penn to illustrate them.

Phenomenology accounts for the information which psychoanalysts access in conducting their transformational work; perspectivism describes the variety of viewpoints from which psychoanalysts, as well as their patients, consider these phenomena; holism extends perspectivism by studying parts within wholes and wholes within parts; and existentialism provides insights into the common experiences of *being* human—death, responsibility, aloneness, and meaning. These basic philosophical viewpoints allow psychoanalysts to explore the human experience as affected from within, such as childhood trauma or neurobiology; they allow them to consider subjectivity as affected from without, such as by social, historical, and cultural forces. They transcend differences in psychoanalytic theories, encompassing the approaches used by psychoanalytic clinicians of even widely divergent theoretical orientations.

Phenomenology

The term "phenomenology," derived from the Greek *phainomenon*, meaning "appearance," originated in ancient Hindu and Buddhist philosophies. First coined by Johann Heinrich Lambert[11] in 1894, Georg

Wilhelm Friedrich Hegel[12] laid the groundwork for its expansion by subsequent German philosophers, specifically Edmund Husserl[13] and Martin Heidegger.[14] Husserl's potent call to return "back to the things themselves"[15] privileged raw subjective phenomena, the *stuff* of human experience evident in language, behavior, thought, and emotion. Phenomenology features significantly in any clinical psychoanalytic theory precisely because of its emphasis upon the subjective point of view.

Heidegger refers to our human experience as a "clearing." He considers phenomenology a basic and unifying philosophy. Donna Orange, a contemporary psychoanalyst, similarly views it as a "rich source of challenges to our easy inner-outer account of mind, emotion, and motivation."[16] She recommends depth psychotherapists utilize dialectical, paradoxical, and shifting perspectives in listening to seemingly paradoxical patient information. Her viewpoint anticipates perspectivism. Essentially, clinicians, in partnership with their patients, attend to the phenomena patients present. They listen to their words, look at their gestures, observe the drama unfolding between the two parties, and feel tension present, absent, or projected onto some external entity.

I clearly recall my initial impressions of Carlos, Gilda, and Penn, e.g., the phenomenology of their presentations. Carlos' propensity to idealize struck me immediately. He shared the fateful story of his weeping at his daughter's private school and more. In his observable behavior, Carlos appeared poorly dressed for a man of his economic stature. He wore a T-shirt, sweatpants, and sneakers. He smiled broadly, with confidence, eager to begin the re-parenting process he imagined awaited him. No distress was evident. In terms of the phenomena of my own experience, I felt somewhat ill at ease with Carlos. He seemed more prepared to begin our journey than I. Phenomenology consists of the rough collection of sensory experiences, as Husserl suggested. I strive, in describing Carlos so far, to prevent interpreting his appearance or behavior in any way; neither do I interpret mine.

Gilda's presentation completely differed. Her emotional experiences took the lead during our first few minutes together. She expressed sadness as she described her recent termination from her retiring psychoanalyst. She was reserved, cautious, and tentative. Whereas she led with her emotions, I responded to her appearance. She was tall and statuesque. Her olive skin glowed in the dark light of my consulting room.

Emanating more sensuality than sexuality, Gilda dressed conservatively, almost formally, in a dark gray business dress. I received her description of her life situation as if presented in a picture frame: her mourning of her last psychoanalyst, her worry about her work situation, and her "terrible" childhood. I felt stricken by her sadness, which, fortunately, broke the intensity of my magnetic-like attraction to her. Equally intense was my desire to rescue her. She was the consummate damsel in distress.

My recollection of the phenomena emanating from Penn, then a young man, is vague. It has been many years now. Lean and delicate, his anxiety propelled him forward in the consulting room armchair. He displayed more anxiety than any specific mood state. He feared failure. Penn wanted quick solutions to his problems. He struggled with *being*, having already, even at his young age, become over-identified with its opposite, *doing*.

A noteworthy deviation from the philosophies to follow, please notice, again, how my descriptions of the three patients include *my* sensory perceptions of them intermixed with their verbal reports. With Penn, for example, I felt tempted to link together the rapidity of his speech, his describing feeling "always on the run," and his devotion to *doing* over *being* into an interpretation of some sort. But any deeper consideration of meaning strays beyond the confines of phenomenology. The initial stage of any psychoanalytic encounter consists of an observation of phenomena. It is a gathering of the experience of patients, from them and from me. These initial sessions exemplify the relevance of phenomenology, which applies equally to every session, and to every moment within every session.

Perspectivism

Perspectivism is a sibling to phenomenology, offering a means for parsing the phenomenological, subjective phenomena just described. It considers multiple points of view. Baruch Spinoza,[17] with his risky substance dualism, paid a heavy price for his use of perspectivism. Ejected first from Judaism and later from Christianity, his observation that human subjectivity represents just one possible perspective alienated him from both religions. Most of his peers believed the transcendent soul manifested, in part, as human subjectivity. Spinoza, with his devotion to monism, disagreed. He considered subjectivity just one angle. His aspect dualism, in direct opposition to substance dualism, led to his repeated banishment. Perspectivism traces its earliest roots in ancient Greek philosophy, but Friedrich Nietzsche first coined the term, writing "it is precisely facts that do not exist, only interpretations ..."[18] By interpretations, he meant perspectives.

When purely in the role of *Lover* waiting for patients to free associate, or when, as *Exorcist* or *Critic*, drawing patients into discussion, depth psychotherapists ultimately bring alternative perspectives into view. The number of possible angles—influenced by history, culture, socioeconomic status, educational level, and more—is immeasurable. Such complexity increases when including patients, psychoanalysts, and the relationship between them into the mix. Psychoanalytic theories of mind or practice are essentially perspectives in themselves.

Some psychoanalytic scholars view perspectivism with ambivalence. Contemporary depth psychotherapist Richard Chessick, for example, worries it invites an excessive "tolerance of differing points of view presented by prestigious or otherwise qualified individuals [and also encourages] a relativism in which one idea is as good as another."[19] Other psychoanalytic scholars prefer to qualify the word "perspectivism" with other words for clarity. Aron coins the phrase "relational-perspectivism"[20] to highlight how perspectives are co-created by patients and their psychoanalysts. Proposing precisely the same idea of co-participation, Hoffman prefers the phrase "social constructivism."[21] Orange likes "perspectival realism,"[22] acknowledging the viewpoints of all parties—not just psychoanalysts and their patients. She fears memories, perceptions, and feelings might be viewed as constructs rather than real to the involved parties. Her use of the word "realism" emphasizes patients' perception of reality. Because I limit this exploration to clinical work only, these disagreements regarding perspectivism, or the proposed modifications with words like realism or constructionism, become of more academic than pragmatic relevance. I propose perspectivism as a foundational philosophy for clinical psychoanalysis precisely because it acknowledges *all* possible points of view, even the scrappy disputes just noted.

In the final analysis, most psychoanalytic scholars endorse perspectivism. Aron, for example, considers psychoanalytic work as requiring "the analyst's openness to new perspectives, a commitment to take other perspectives seriously, and a refusal to view any interpretation as complete or any meaning as exhaustive."[23] Who could argue against the idea that, clinically, patients present their own perspectives, depth psychotherapists similarly have theirs, and unique perspectives emerge from their relationship? Stephen Mitchell, who initiated relational psychoanalysis, acknowledges perspectivism's "important contribution."[24] Paralleling my efforts to seek commonalities between different theoretical perspectives, Henry Smith views perspectivism as fundamental to psychoanalytic encounters, regardless of clinicians' theoretical preferences, writing:

> I believe we would find each of us certain of the ultimate truth of an observation at some points and thoroughly aware of the limits on our own perspective at others, as we struggle with the subjective components in both the patient's and our own minds at work.[25]

Having defined perspectivism and offered examples of its appearance in the recent psychoanalytic literature, I apply the concept to the three patients. I utilize two narrowly focused lenses: cultural factors and psychoanalytic theories due to space constraints. I rely upon ideas promoted by Wallerstein, who considers psychoanalytic theory as offering a "diversity of explanatory metaphors,"[26] and by Greenberg, who refers to them as "controlling fictions."[27] I am not endorsing random eclecticism. Instead, I suggest that depth psychotherapists carefully match their use of metaphors, fictions, or models to each specific patient. Here are some examples of how I used perspectivism in my work with these three individuals:

Carlos' Latino heritage plays a major role in his view of the world. He proclaims its influence on him with pride, considering himself "a paragon of machismo." Rather pathetically, Carlos dismisses other stereotypes of Latin culture, like warmth, softness, sensuality, and emotionality. Carlos lives the life of the macho man. His impoverished early childhood experience, his brothers' involvement in crime and gangs, and the geography of his ghetto-like childhood homes, shaped his personal experience as much as his Latin blood. Psychological factors, in addition to cultural ones, contributed to Carlos' deep sense of personal insecurity. More than the economic impoverishment, Carlos endured a frightening, lonely childhood. He witnessed his father abusing his mother, was victimized by his older half-brothers, and was repeatedly displaced. These traumata devastated his sense of self. In order to protect the resultant vulnerability, he developed narcissistic compensatory mechanisms. Where others might feel weak or exposed, Carlos never would. In like manner, his tendency to view himself, and certain others (like me) in idealized, grandiose terms, also shields him.

On rare occasions, I encountered the originally wounded boy, the crying mess, and the frightened kid. Michael Balint, a key figure in British object relations theory, considers these moments "a regression in the interest of progression," a chance for patients like Carlos to experience a "new beginning."[28] So my capacity to contain and to hold Carlos' experiences of sadness, loss, and terror during these moments allowed healing to occur. The lonely boy became less lonely; the terror became more manageable. In my role of *Lover*, I provided sanctuary for the fragile self he worked so vehemently to hide. At times, my role as *Exorcist* allowed him to demonstrate to me, in real time, the persistent, deep feeling of loneliness. As *Critic*, I introduced Carlos to these ideas over time, further enhancing his understanding of self and his perceptions of others.

Another example of the unique nature of each sociocultural context, Gilda descended from Greek Orthodox roots. Not religious herself, her parents were married in the Church, immigrated from Greece in the early twentieth century, and Greek was the primary language spoken in the family home. Gilda, although speaking with a slight Greek accent herself, felt little overt racism as a "foreigner." However, as a first-generation American, she recalls feeling some alienation from her peers. She felt embarrassed, for example, by her parents' strong accents (when speaking English). Sexual harassment was, unfortunately, a consistent part of her experience from adolescence onward. She felt objectified by others, and here I refer to people outside her family circle. And the attention was not limited to men. While serving as a teaching assistant in American history, one of her female professors made a sexual advance toward her. Gilda politely declined, but the situation was awkward. These cultural and gender-based perspectives sculpted Gilda's subjective world.

Gilda's psychological development differs from Carlos' in an almost mathematically perfect fashion. Whereas he externalized vulnerability, she internalized it. She interpreted the abuse by her father, the neglect by her mother, and even the sexual objectification as evidence of her unworthiness. Instead of developing Carlos' Teflon-like shell, Gilda felt terrible about herself—insecure, inadequate, unworthy. Much later in our work together, Gilda accessed rage at, first, the molestation and, later, the sexual assault to which she was subjected. For many months, however, discussions of these traumatic events were met by Gilda's guiltily feeling responsible for them. The physical assault she endured at the work party aggravated these internal dynamics even more. The PTSD was intensified by her propensity toward internal attacks. It took months for Gilda to access her rage at the adults who abused her during her childhood. In like manner, it took months for her to access rage at her attackers and at her employer for failing to support her after the assault.

Penn's sociocultural background offers less evidence of neglect or objectification. Here, again, an opportunity exists to explore more subtle cultural differences. Penn was reared in the comfort of an upper-class Caucasian environment, embraced by the security of the dominant culture of his time. The primary cultural perspective, then, consists of the Protestant, even Calvinist tendencies of his (ironically) Jewish family background. Little attention was paid to Judaism. Neither Penn nor his parents attended Temple. He did not pass through the ritual of the Bar Mitzvah. However, his father expected him to follow in his, and his grandfather's, medical footsteps. Moreover, every bit of worth and value in life rested in academic and economic achievement. *Being* had little value; *doing* was everything. Penn ingested the value system hook, line, and sinker.

Coincidentally, the psychoanalytic perspective on Penn follows closely from the cultural one, and it includes the oft-misunderstood concept of the Oedipus complex. Falsely interpreted as meaning children wishing to literally have sex with their opposite-gendered parent, the Oedipus complex actually describes the transition from infancy to adulthood. Infants tend to develop dyadically, that is, intensive two-person relationships with their caregivers. They bond most with a single caregiver, and then they bask in the glow of feeling like the *only* apple in their caregiver's eyes. The Oedipus complex, roughly speaking, consists of the transition from this immersive, one-on-one experience, into broader interpersonal contexts. A gradual weaning occurs during which the infant, and then the toddler, slowly, and painfully realizes the presence of others beyond the blissful sphere of the initial party of two. After the destruction of the illusion of perfect two-ness, children gradually adapt to configurations of three, four, or more others. They become part of a family, of larger groups, and ultimately of society. The loss of that exclusive love is immeasurable. Some, like Lacan,[29] think we spend the rest of our lives re-seeking it. Our ultimate desire consists of the wish for unconditional love. The Oedipus complex oversimplifies the evolution from dyadic to triadic relations and beyond. In addition, it suffers from its tragic arc and its inherent sexism.

I borrow one additional and key psychoanalytic concept, from Fairbairn, to enhance readers' understanding of Penn. Fairbairn thought that—and I consider this one of the most important contributions to the psychoanalytic opus—infants and toddlers adapt to neglect, abuse, or a mistreatment by their parents by adopting a negative self-image. In order to maintain their parents as god-like figures, they consider themselves "bad." Fairbairn proposed that, when thus let down, infants unconsciously assume blame. They sacrifice their own self-valuation to maintain the sanctity of the caregivers. (Obviously, the concept applies to Gilda's and Carlos' psychology as well.) The creation of the unconscious internal world, Fairbairn argues, occurs as a means of retaining the real external, parental figures' crucially powerful status. Meanwhile, "dynamic structures,"[30] consisting of images of self (as bad or good) and of other (as persecuting or supportive) develop. Another key concept, Fairbairn considered these images interlinked. Your images of self and other are always related to one another. Fairbairn termed the negative other-to-self-component of the dynamic structure the "internal saboteur."[31]

For Penn, both the Oedipus complex and Fairbairn's psychodynamic model explain what haunts him. In a sense, Penn never completely transcended into adulthood. He is stuck, unconsciously, in a perpetual competition with his father. The mere possibility of failure is felt as catastrophic. It would mean, unconsciously for him, complete disaster, abandonment, a relinquishing of even the remote hope of being loved. At the same time, Penn internalized the neglect by his parents into a dynamic structure consisting of a highly critical internal other assaulting his intensely negative sense of self. He constantly runs to escape it, to free himself from terrific feelings of aloneness and abandonment. He seeks achievement he falsely hopes will bring him love. Much of my work with Penn consists of helping him face the original, primitive loss, and to experience the futility of his search for repair through the endless, compulsive pursuit of accomplishment.

Holism

First coined by Jan Christian Smuts,[32] the term *holism* refers to a philosophy describing the functioning of complex systems. Specifically, it encompasses dynamic connections between parts and wholes. Holism views complicated organizational entities, like human subjectivities, as irreducible to interacting parts like the superego torturing the ego. No one part can be considered in isolation from others. The Hungarian intellectual Arthur Koestler coined the word *holon*[33] to describe an entity existing simultaneously as a whole and a part. He argued that, in living and social organizations, holons exist as simultaneously self-contained wholes relating to their subordinate parts, and as self-contained parts relating to wholes. Referring to a "holarchy of holons," Koestler describes the human organism as:

> A hierarchy of self-regulating holons which function (a) as autonomous wholes in supra-ordination to their parts, (b) as dependent parts in subordination to controls on higher levels, (c) in coordination with their local environment.[34]

It follows logically that our topic of interest, human subjectivities, may *not* be accurately defined as indivisible, self-contained units with independent existences. Koestler elaborates, noting that separate entities are:

> nowhere found in Nature or society, just as we nowhere find absolute wholes. Instead of separateness and independence, there is cooperation and inter-dependence, running through the whole gamut, from physical symbiosis to the cohesive bonds of the swarm, hive, shoal, flock, herd, family, society.[35]

Several psychoanalytic scholars specifically apply holism to the field. Jonathon Lear[36] believes Freud embraced *"psychological* holism." Patients' verbal reports, or nonverbal behaviors, he believes, exist within a web of wishes, desires, and other conscious and unconscious forces embodied within a living organism. Contemporary psychoanalyst Lewis Kirshner[37] uses holism to describe the dynamic relationship between patients and psychoanalysts. He describes the ego, or self, as "more than the ensemble of these phenomena, just as a melody is not an entity to which musical notes refer, but exists only in the indissolubility of its elements."[38] Barnaby Barratt describes how psychoanalysis consists of co-participants reflecting on their discourse—another type of holism. He writes of the need to think about such interactions "without lapsing into an outmoded Cartesian dualism that disrespects what we now know to be the holism of what I will call the 'bodymind'."[39]

Several psychoanalytic scholars, myself among them, use holism to achieve greater cohesion in psychoanalytic models of mind and practice. S. Montana Katz believes the use of metaphors, on the one hand, and the capacity for interpersonal communication, on the other, comprise both parts and wholes of psychoanalytic processes. Regarding metaphors themselves, she believes they provide a "vast overlap of sinews across persons [which] affords inter- and intra-subjective awareness and exchange." Holism provides a potentially unifying, robust psychoanalytic model unattainable by other, more linear ones, and thereby allowing "human access to both the internal and the external worlds," she writes, adding that holism offers "the potential to articulate the underlying similarities and differences between analytic perspectives and therefore to broaden and deepen understanding of theoretical principles and clinical techniques."[40] Jerome Appelbaum also finds holism a bridge between psychoanalysts' theoretical differences, noting how,

> Unlike a jigsaw puzzle where the individual pieces can only fit together in a single particular manner to form a whole, psychoanalysis can be analogized as an erector set where the same pieces can form different wholes ... [just like the way in which] the protagonists in a narrative story might have been considered as differently related.[41]

In the same vein, Steven Stern utilizes holism to explain how psychoanalysts can tailor psychoanalytic models and methods to specific patients. He alludes to psychoanalysts commonly mistaking parts for wholes, and vice versa. He laments their tendency to "enshrine a particular principle or set of principles of therapeutic action implied by a given theory as the foundational and universal path to psychoanalytic transformation," adding in italics, *"we don't tend to think of the analytic relationship more holistically."*[42] Marcia Cavell uses the phrase "the holism of the mental," referring to relations between mental phenomena and the outside world. She describes human beings as "creatures who, through our interactions with other creatures in a world we share in common, come to mean something by our utterances."[43] Melvin Bornstein considers holism central to contemporary psychoanalytic thinking, writing:

> In an era of pluralism, holism has become more integrated into psychoanalysis. Self, person, and personality are concepts that can more comfortably exist alongside systemic entities such as drives, ego, id, defense, conflict, and so forth. The humane experience of psychoanalysis based on the dignity of human beings and the achievement of self-awareness, creativity, love, and the joy of living can be brought more easily into the clinical model.[44]

Additionally, holism allows for the layering of unique perspectives. It differs from but also extends perspectivism. The complex influence of ethnicity, for example, finds an organizational home within holism. So do the complicated psychoanalytic ideas of transference and countertransference. Holism addresses the unfortunate fragmentation existing in contemporary clinical psychoanalysis. Rather than choosing between drive-structural or relational-structural theories,[45] depth psychotherapists can improvise depending upon the phenomenology of patients. The anger in an extremely sexually charged sixteen-year-old adolescent may require a clinician to incorporate drive theory and interpersonal models. Holism invites such unique combinations.

Psychoanalytic field theories also incorporate holism. These models consider psychoanalytic couples, what psychoanalyst Douglas Ingram calls their "signature,"[46] as unique. William and Madeline Baranger[47] and Katz[48] offer generalized field theories. Other similar theories include Robert Galatzer-Levy's[49] dynamic systems theory, Michael Miller's[50] complex dynamic interacting systems model, William Coburn's[51] multiple interpenetrating systems theory, and Robert Stolorow's[52] phenomenological contextualism. These encompass parts within wholes—the individuals within the psychoanalytic relationship; and they also encompass wholes by considering the broader context of the relationship itself. In sum, holism describes complex, multi-layered patterns inexplicable by other foundational philosophies.

I limit my application of holism in the cases of Carlos, Gilda, and Penn to *only* transference and countertransference (also to prevent this volume from running thousands of pages). By transference, I mean any outside-the-room interpersonal pattern mapped onto psychoanalytic relationships by patients. These include ones originating from childhood, such as unresolved anger toward parents, or any *transferred* relational patterns, including contemporaneous relationships. Transference could include, for example, wives projecting anger at their husbands onto their depth psychotherapists. Countertransference refers to the same phenomena but in reverse: They consist of the relational patterns—with their concomitant emotions, attitudes, and cognitions—projected by depth psychotherapists onto their patients.

Beginning with Carlos, the transference pattern, as noted previously, consisted of a remarkable idealization broken by a sudden, abrupt devaluation when I fell ill. Holism is relevant because Carlos' traumatic history created the idealization process. It defended him against feeling the sense of inadequacy simmering beneath the surface. When my medical leave abruptly ended our meetings, I unintentionally stimulated Carlos' darkest fears—of abandonment, of not mattering. In this specific instance, his immediate, adult experience mimicked his infantile one. My illness created loss, trauma, and indemnity. It blew Carlos' mind. His initial reaction was flight. As you know, Carlos began working with me in a state of blissful safety. He sought help because he broke into tears in public, feeling the stark differences between his daughter's school experience and his. He initially avoided any feelings of vulnerability by wrapping both of us up into the warm blanket of his idealism. Because of my own childhood injuries, I enjoyed the glow for several months. Heinz Kohut considers this a twinship transference.[53] Carlos' sense of "aren't we both awesome" allowed him to feel comfortable in the relationship with me.

Also, he needed the "holding environment," a replication of a parenting experience suggested by psychoanalyst Donald Winnicott. Only after passing through such a safe, rapport-building environment could Carlos regress in a manner inviting him to address his deep emotional wounds.

During those brief periods in which Carlos wept, asked me to parent him, and pled for my help, the transference inverted. I remained idealized, but Carlos descended into infantile pain. He relived the acute feelings of terror, abandonment, aloneness, and loss of his early childhood years. These moments were intense, exposing emotional states hidden from consciousness for decades. He shared memories that accompanied these emotional states, like the hours alone with his brothers, missing his mother, his father's physical abuse of his mother, and his loneliness. As I will explain in subsequent chapters, these regressive periods seemed to foment the most change in Carlos. They provided what Franz Alexander called "corrective emotional experience."[54] Holism appears in the many levels of the transference–countertransference configuration with Carlos.

As expected, these configurations developed differently in my work with Gilda. As with all patients, my work with her elicited unique aspects of my own personality—some positive, some negative. Each psychoanalytic dyad assumes a life of its own. Beginning with my countertransference, her open, exposed, yearning-like presentation elicited a desire to rescue what I have felt for few others. The physical attraction for her aggravated such rescue fantasies. Until she was injured, I kept my desires within reasonable bounds. However, after the assault, I struggled to maintain boundaries. Her dissociative episodes triggered my moving from worry to emotional over-involvement. Interestingly, I began experiencing symptoms parallel to Gilda's. She went through a period of insomnia; I, too, had difficulty sleeping. She felt terror at her life unraveling; I felt frightened of failing her.

At times, attraction to patients results from an unconscious seductiveness on their part; at other times, it has nothing to do with the patient. In the situation with Gilda, I take full responsibility. I do not believe she, consciously or unconsciously, behaved seductively. The combination of my natural attraction to her, and the power differential related to my social role, led me into an over-involvement I describe later. No overt sexual involvement ever occurred. However, my level of caring for her, and my way of verbally and nonverbally expressing it, exceeded the bounds of the professional relationship. Ultimately, we managed to utilize my loss of navigation as a learning experience for her (as well as for me).

Gilda, like Carlos, displayed some idealization of me. It lacked the grandiosity characteristic of Carlos. It was innocent. Gilda placed the vulnerable core of her being—so elusive in my work with Carlos—directly into my arms. She trusted me. She tested me a bit, at first, most likely because of the transition from her prior long-term psychoanalyst to me. However, she fairly quickly became invested in me, and in our relationship. We were strongly connected by the time she was attacked. After the assault, our relationship entered a one-year period of problematic enactments on my part. In the way of a further introduction, Gilda interpreted my emotional over-involvement as a *real* repair. She felt our relationship transcended the doctor–patient one. Her perception was correct. I had, at some point along the way, lost my professional authority. If *narcissism* refers to an over-involvement with the self, then *masochism* refers to persons who undervalue themselves. Over time, Gilda and I fell into an oscillating sadomasochistic pattern.

Before that time, the transference and countertransference relationships assumed the typical motifs I reported earlier. Essentially, and fearing being repetitive now, Gilda became more regressed and needy. Some of her behaviors, particularly the psychogenic fugue states, invited me into an almost supernatural role. I felt responsible for her life. I intervened in ways I rarely did. I contacted her psychopharmacologist to coordinate the medication. I reached out to her daughter to, in a sense, deputize her during that particularly dangerous period. Most significantly, I recommended Gilda attend sessions six days a week. I offered such frequent appointments because I feared for her life. I considered it preferable to inpatient psychiatric hospitalization, which I consider an absolutely last course of action—a holding pen for patients whose suicidal actions, psychotic states, or other emergency mental conditions require constant monitoring.

After the year involving troubling enactments described in later chapters, Gilda and I decided, together, to reduce session frequency. The intensity of the post-traumatic reaction lessened. She required less interaction. We actively discussed reducing the meetings and how she might react. Nonetheless, once instituted, Gilda found the loss difficult to bear. Her relationship with others in her life, including her daughter, had been strained by her acute post-traumatic distress. I had become her only outlet, her only friend. The transition allows me to elaborate upon what I meant by sadomasochistic oscillations. As I returned to the usual role of psychoanalytic psychotherapist, Gilda felt abandoned. She was also angry. I fear I had, in a sense, abused her during that period of intensive work. Her father's partner's abuse was overt. However, and like him and other abusers, I gained from Gilda's affection and attention. While I certainly attended to her closely out of concern, I equally enacted my own needs.

Here, the sadomasochistic theme emerges with greater clarity. While reacting to my pulling back from her, she expressed her hurt and rage. She accused me of behaving unprofessionally. In many ways, she was correct. At those points, I became the small, inadequate party. She became the persecutor. In contrast, when I occupied the caregiving role, I was the powerful party, and she was the weak, needy care-receiver. While we worked together to return the relationship to its proper bounds, these roles switched back and forth—sometimes even within a single session. Fortunately, after an equilibrium returned, we resumed the depth psychoanalytic work for several additional years.

Meanwhile, consider the metaphor of the tight-rope walker as an analogy for balancing personal caring and psychoanalytic interventions.[55] In brief, psychodynamic psychotherapists walk along a tight wire balancing their real emotional involvement with patients with their devotion to professionally facilitating transformation. In the period immediately following Gilda's assault. I fell from the high wire. And when her crisis period passed, I readjusted the professional relationship. This painful example of the transference and countertransference with Gilda uncomfortably demonstrates the holism, the layered parts within the wholes of any psychoanalytic relationship. In my work with her, so many levels interacted—including, initially, my attraction to her, her innocent trust in me, and later, that fragile fault-line erupting into a full-fledged earthquake when she regressed, and I became over-involved. We both enacted features of our traumatic histories. My crossing boundaries through over-involvement and excessive self-disclosure added another layer to the already impasto-like depth of our involvement with one another.

Given that Penn had, overall, less childhood trauma than either Carlos or Gilda, the transference and countertransference configurations invading our relationship were less complicated. I closely identified with Penn from the start. I understood his competition with his father. I understood the price one pays for overemphasizing doing over being. I recall clearly seeing him, all those many decades ago, as a younger version of myself. The transference relationship mirrored the countertransference one. Penn looked up to me. Our relationship has been spared any significant narcissistic or masochistic enactments. Instead, it stayed within proper professional boundaries throughout. Neither Carlos' flight from me nor Gilda's iatrogenic, one-year regression infected our journey.

Nonetheless, at times, Penn's desperate, infantile level of competition with his father entered his relationship with me. Thomas Szasz defines psychoanalytic work as consisting of the analysis of the contractual elements of the relationships with patients, specifically "of the therapeutic situation and of extra-analytic situations in which the patient plays a significant part."[56] The meta-commentary on the work with Carlos and Gilda became most meaningful, and ultimately transformational, during the dramatic enactments just noted. My relationship with Penn lacked drama. I empathized with his level of anxiety, which, at times, became intense. Even now, I feel great sympathy for his chronic inability to feel adequate despite his professional accomplishments. For Penn, the number of degrees, awards, professorships, or publications lifts his spirits only briefly. His biological vulnerability, greatly aggravated by childhood trauma, left him injured and wounded. When acute, the inflammation of his emotional vulnerability overshadows any of his "merely mortal" accomplishments.

During the darkest of his moments journeying with me, Penn ironically expressed envy at my own achievements. It was fascinating to witness his inability to conceive of *me* experiencing the same emptiness. Here, Penn's perception demonstrates both projection and idealization. He imagined my achievements brought me the pride he thought it would give him—a form of projection. His belief that it bolstered me (in a way elusive to him) represented an idealization. These transference and countertransference themes unfolded gently, and unlike they had with either Carlos or Gilda. My focus remains on helping him experience *being* in a safe, soothing, and comfortable way. However, much like what occurred with Carlos and Gilda, Penn achieves the most growth when he descends into his deep feelings of inadequacy.

It is at those points he has no choice but to immerse himself in the childhood pain, vent it, and bring it into the light. He re-experiences the discomfort in a safer, healing environment, each time enhancing his capacity to *be*.

At times, I become frustrated with Penn's glacial-like forward movement. The difference between his self-perception and the world's perception of him, remains striking. I consider the problem mine, not his. I strive to keep the trauma that shaped his character in mind. I think of his struggles to internalize others' positive perceptions of him as a means of providing comfort for himself. Nonetheless, I sometimes became impatient. An example of the power of the unconscious mind, Penn noticed this streak of annoyance well before I did. Penn closely attends to my emotional states. My occasional irritation lights up his inner sense of unworthiness. At these times, he feels *he* is failing *me*. For some years now, we review this dance whenever he returns for sets of sessions. A painful process, for sure, but these active, real-time encounters, further facilitate his moving toward overcoming discomfort with being. The benefit is obviously *not* because Penn wishes to please me. Each time we enter this specific dynamic, my frustration versus his need to please, Penn bears the pain. He understands and emotionally experiences, in real time, the futility of his striving to please the other. Gradually, the control of the internal saboteur lessens its grip. On rare occasions, Penn becomes angry at me. He rightfully confronts me with *my* expectations—one of the clearest indications of his growth. Historically, his response was singular and rigid: *He* must be wrong, and he must work harder to "perform." Over the course of our many years of knowing one another, Penn has, overall, grown more self-confident. He feels less controlled by his compulsions. More times than ever before, Penn appreciates the *experience* of his life, seeing himself, sometimes only fleetingly, as a thriving, loving person rather than a machine of production.

Existentialism

Many consider Soren Kierkegaard[57] the first existentialist despite him never having formally used the term. Kierkegaard believed Christians must choose their faith freely, and therein lies the emphasis on freedom characteristic of existentialism. In the Denmark of his era, status as a Christian came with citizenship. Kierkegaard extended his ideas of "choosing faith" beyond the theological. He thought individuals retain responsibility for giving meaning to their lives. Subsequent philosophers contributed to the existential opus, with Nietzsche, Fyodor Dostoyevsky, Heidegger, Martin Buber, Albert Camus, and Jean-Paul Sartre among the most significant. Sartre's classic idea of existence preceding essence emphasizes *being* and free choice—arguably taking freedom too far. In other words, and a radical proposition from which he himself backed away from later in his life, you *entirely* choose your life's path. This diametrically opposes the essentialist position, which suggests your path is determined by God, DNA, culture, or other external forces. Heidegger introduced concepts such as *authenticity*, meaning living with a true sense of self, other, and purpose, as well as *thrownness*, referring to the elements of being in which you lack choice, such as where you were born. Ludwig Binswanger[58] brought existential ideas specifically to psychiatry and psychotherapy, as did Karl Jaspers[59] and, more recently, Irwin Yalom.[60]

Many psychoanalysts consider existential philosophy central to their clinical work. Burston[61] believes existentialism "stresses that every individual's way of 'being-in-the-world' is unique, and that the meanings that individuals create and confer on existence are a product of individual values, priorities, and decisions." George Atwood, Stolorow, and Orange[62] describe how their own traumatic experiences keep them "continuingly self-reflective and ever phenomenological, contextual, and perspectival, open to new possibilities of understanding yet to be discovered" when working clinically. By embracing the fundamental and constitutive role of relatedness in creating subjective experience, they argue, their work extends existential philosophy. Jon Mills[63] also considers existential points of view as foundational, describing how they "complement psychoanalytic discourse, thus providing a fecundity of overlap in conceptual thought and practice that the relational schools have been increasingly acknowledging over the past two decades."

Arguably the most significant proponent of combining existentialism and psychoanalysis, Robert Stolorow,[64] believes various life trauma, namely existential experiences, inevitably impact the experiences of psychoanalysts and patients alike. He writes,

On one hand, emotional experience is inseparable from the contexts of attunement and mal-attunement in which it is felt, and painful emotional experiences become enduringly traumatic in the absence of an intersubjective context within which they can be held and integrated. On the other hand, emotional trauma is built into the basic constitution of human existence.[65]

Hoffman[66] critiques the CBT approaches and the neurosciences for their inadequacy in understanding human experiences. Many practitioners find these subjects appealing, he thinks, because they offer the illusion of understanding. They minimize the daunting responsibility psychoanalysts feel as they encounter new and ambiguous experiences in patients who are free agents.

No surprise, then, existentialism as a philosophy, and as it applies to depth psychotherapy, places great value on freedom. It considers authenticity a primary virtue. Whatever has brought patients to seek help from psychoanalysts, existential themes linger. Much like the serenity prayer preached in Alcoholics Anonymous (AA), depth psychotherapists help patients make more informed, clear choices, while paradoxically facilitating their surrendering to the forces over which they have no control. In addition to greeting the phenomena their patients emanate, and considering the holistic layering of their experiences, they also honor the existential sense of disorientation or confusion as patients face an apparently meaningless world. An excerpt from A.E. Houseman's poem, "The laws of God, the laws of man," captures the humbling feeling well:

> I, a stranger and afraid
> In a world I never made.[67]

After escorting their patients into their consulting rooms, psychoanalysts begin an unmapped journey. Carlos, Gilda, and Penn, in many ways, struggled to make sense of the worlds they never made. Of the three, Carlos showed the least awareness of existential themes. He rarely, if ever, wondered about the meaning of life. Instead, he immersed himself in the quest for money. It symbolized something immensely important to him. And yet, satisfaction continually eluded him.

Something deeper beckons him. In contrast, brilliant Gilda never lost her search for meaning. She looked for answers in literature and philosophy; she inquired into realms of history. Part of her reaction to the assault involved confrontation with death. She may well have been killed during the attack—a reality never lost upon her.

Ironically, Penn struggles the most existentially, and in all four dimensions that Yalom identifies as central to depth psychotherapy—aloneness, responsibility, meaninglessness, and death. Penn felt responsible for achieving, for supporting his family, and for caring for his patients well before he finished medical school. No matter how much his wife, children, patients, colleagues, relatives, and friends showered him with admiration and love, Penn never lost his sense of aloneness. His mother's constant fury left him feeling fearful throughout his early childhood. The anxiety deprived him of the basic sense of security of which Erik Erikson[68] writes. Death, for Penn, framed life. He chose orthopedic surgery because it allowed him to help younger, injured persons. On the rare occasions he encountered bone cancers, he sighed with relief after referring them to his oncology colleagues who thereafter assumed responsibility for their care. Penn's conscious avoidance of death betrayed a deeper influence by it. Along these same lines, and describing his experiences with opium, the poet Jean Cocteau writes:

> Everything we do in life, including love, is done in an express train traveling toward death. To smoke opium is to leave the train while in motion; it is to be interested in something other than life and death.[69]

No wonder alcoholism and substance abuse remain the primary mental health disorders around the globe. What is Cocteau's point? Life and death always run like ice-cold streams beneath our conscious minds. For him, opium stopped him from shivering, and eliminated the sense of immersion altogether. Although only Carlos overtly struggled with addictions, specifically to tranquilizers and alcohol, all three patients wrestled with existential issues. In summary, then, psychoanalysts begin with the phenomena presented to them. They then utilize perspectivism to explore their patients' phenomenological presentations from various angles. Holism adds a layering capacity to perspectivism, providing a language for articulating the transference and countertransference. How? Because while the involved parties might be discussing ambivalence about a marriage, they are, at the same time, engaged in an interpersonal enactment of unconscious themes on another layer. Finally, existentialism highlights the basic life themes—death being a rather prominent one—which constantly haunt the human mind. In the next chapter, I turn to the intricacies of psychoanalytic theorizing, a holistic exploration *par excellence*. As you will see, these parallel the evolution of thought in the Western world, from modernist to postmodernist, from structuralist to post-structuralist, and from Newtonian to Einsteinian physics.

Notes

1. Wilber, K. (2000). *Integral Psychology*. Boston, MA: Shambala.
2. Foucault, M. (1963). *The Birth of the Clinic: An Archeology of Medical Perception*. A. Sheridan (Trans.). New York, NY: Routledge.
3. Einstein, A. (2005). *Relativity: The Special and General Theory*. Robert W. Lawson (Trans.). New York, NY: Pi Press.
4. Heisenberg, W. (2000). *Physics and Philosophy*. New York, NY: Penguin.
5. Nagel, E., & Newman, N.R. (2001). *Godel's Proof*. New York, NY: New York Universities Press.
6. Wittgenstein, L. (2009). *Philosophical Investigations*. G.E.M. Anscombe, P.M.S. Hacker & Joachim Schulte (Trans.). New York, NY: Blackwell. (Original work published in 1953.)
7. Kuhn, T. (2012). *The Structure of Scientific Paradigms*. Chicago, IL: University of Chicago Press. (Original work published in 1962.)
8. Derrida, J. *Writing and Difference*. Alan Bass (Trans.). London: Routledge.
9. Gadamer, H.-G. (1991). *Truth and Method*. New York, NY: Crossroads Publishing.
10. Darwin, C. (1998). *The Origin of the Species*. London: Wordsworth Editions Limited. (Original work published in 1859.)
11. Lambert, J.H. (1894). *Anmerkungen und Zusätze zur Entwerfung der Land- und Himmelscharten*. Leipzig: Verlag Von Wilhem Engelmann. (Original work published in 1772.)
12. Hegel, G.W.F. (2009). *Phenomenology of Spirit*. A.V. Miller (Trans.). London: Oxford University Press. (Original work published in 1807.)

13. Husserl, E. (2012). Ideas: *General Introduction to Pure Phenomenology.* W.R.B. Gibson (Trans.). New York, NY: Routledge. (Original work published in 1931.)

14. Heidegger, M. (2008). *Being and Time.* John Macquarrie and Edward Robinson (Trans.). New York, NY: HarperCollins. (Original work published in 1927.)

15. Ibid., p. 168.

16. Orange, D. (2002). There is no outside. *Psychoanalytic Psychology,* 19(4): 686–700.

17. Spinoza, B. (1996). *Ethics.* E. Curley (Trans.). New York, NY: Penguin. (Original work published in 1677.)

18. Nietzsche, F. (2002). *Human, All Too Human.* R.J. Hollingdale (Trans.). Cambridge: Cambridge University Press. (Original work published in 1878.)

19. Chessick, R.D. (1997). Perspectivism, constructivism, and empathy in psychoanalysis. *Journal of the American Academy of Psychoanalysis and Dynamic Psychotherapy,* 25(3): 373–398, p. 383.

20. Aron, L. (1992). Interpretation as expression of the analyst's subjectivity. *Psychoanalytic Dialogues,* 2(4): 475–507.

21. Hoffman, I.Z. (1991). Discussion: toward a social-constructivist view of the psychoanalytic situation. *Psychoanalytic Dialogues,* 1(1): 74–105.

22. Orange, D.M. (2002). There is no outside. *Psychoanalytic Psychology,* 19(4): 686–700.

23. Aron, L. (1992). Interpretation as expression of the analyst's subjectivity. *Psychoanalytic Dialogues,* 2(4): 475–507, p. 481n.

24. Mitchell, S.A. (1995). Interaction in the Kleinian and interpersonal traditions. *Contemporary Psychoanalysis,* 31: 65.

25. Smith, H.F. (2001). Obstacles to integration: another look at why we talk past each other. *Psychoanalytic Psychology,* 18(3): 485–514.

26. Wallerstein, R.S. (2013). Metaphor in psychoanalysis and clinical data. In S. Montana Katz (Ed.), *Metaphor and Field: Common Ground, Common Language, and the Future of Psychoanalysis* (pp. 22–38). New York, NY: Routledge, p. 36.

27. Greenberg, J.R. (2015). Therapeutic action and the analyst's responsibility. *Journal of the American Psychoanalytic Association,* 63: 15–32. doi: 10.1177/0003065114561861, p. 17.

28. Balint, M. (1979). *The Basic Fault.* New York, NY: Brunner/Mazel.

29. Lacan, J. (2008). *My Teaching.* D. Macey (Trans.). New York, NY: Verso.

30. Fairbairn, W.R.D. (1952). *Psychoanalytic Studies of the Personality*. London: Routledge, p. 377.

31. Ibid., p. 374.

32. Smuts, J.C. (1986). *Holism and Evolution*. Gouldsboro, ME: Gestalt Journal Press. (Original work published in 1926.)

33. Koestler, A. (1967). *The Ghost in the Machine*. New York NY: Penguin. (Original work published in 1967), p. 45.

34. Ibid., pp. 102–103.

35. Ibid., p. 67.

36. Lear, J. (1993). An interpretation of transference. *International Journal of Psychoanalysis*, 74: 739–755.

37. Kirshner, L.A. (1991). The concept of the self in psychoanalytic theory and its philosophical foundations. *Journal of the American Psychoanalytic Association*, 39: 157–182.

38. Ibid., p. 173.

39. Barratt, B.B. (2010). *The Emergence of Somatic Psychology and Bodymind Therapy*. Basingstoke: Palgrave Macmillan; Barratt, B.B. (2013). Free-associating with the bodymind. *International Forum Psychoanalysis*, 22(3): 161–175.

40. Katz, S.M. (Ed.) (2013). *Metaphor and Field: Common Ground, Common Language, and the Future of Psychoanalysis*. New York, NY: Routledge, p. 132.

41. Appelbaum, J. (2011). Should psychoanalysis become a science? *American Journal of Psychoanalysis*, 71(1): 1–15.

42. Stern, S. (2017). Holistic thinking and therapeutic action: building on Louis Sander's contribution. *Psychoanalytic Dialogues*, 27: 89–103. Doi: 10.1080/10481885.2017.1260959, pp. 90–1.

43. Cavell, M. (1991). The subject of mind. *International Journal of Psychoanalysis*, 72: 141–154.

44. Bornstein, M. (2004). The problem of narcissism in psychoanalytic organizations. *Psychoanalytic Inquiry*, 24(1): 71–85.

45. Greenberg, J.R., & Mitchell, S.A. (1983). *Object Relations in Psychoanalytic Theory*. Cambridge, MA: Harvard University Press.

46. Ingram, D.H. (1994). Poststructuralist interpretation of the psychoanalytic relationship. *Journal of the American Academy of Psychoanalysis*, 22: 175–193, p. 175.

47. Baranger, M., & Baranger, W. (2009). Spiral process and the dynamic field. In L.G. Fiorini (Ed.), *The Work of Confluence: Listening and Interpreting in the*

Psychoanalytic Field (pp. 45–61). London: Karnac. (Original work published in 1979.)

48. Katz, S.M. (Ed.) (2013). *Metaphor and Field: Common Ground, Common Language, and the Future of Psychoanalysis.* New York, NY: Routledge, p. 132.

49. Galatzer-Levy, R.M. (1995). Psychoanalysis and dynamical systems theory: prediction and self-similarity. *Journal of the American Psychoanalytic Association,* 43: 1085–1113.

50. Miller, M.L. (1999). Chaos, complexity, and psychoanalysis. *Psychoanalytic Psychology,* 16: 355–379. Doi: 10.1037/0736-9735.16.3.355.

51. Coburn, W.J. (2002). A world of systems: The role of systemic patterns of experience in the therapeutic process. *Psychoanalytic Inquiry,* 22: 655–677.

52. Stolorow, R.D. (1997). Dynamic, dyadic, intersubjective systems: an evolving paradigm for psychoanalysis. *Psychoanalytic Psychology,* 14: 337–364.

53. Kohut, H. (1979). The two analyses of Mr Z. *International Journal of Psychoanalysis,* 60: 3–27.

54. Alexander, F. (1950). Analysis of the therapeutic factors in psychoanalytic treatment. *Psychoanalytic Quarterly,* 19: 482–500.

55. Karbelnig, A.M. (2018). A perilous high wire act: Framing psychoanalytic relationships with severely traumatized patients. *Psychoanalytic Quarterly,* 87(3): 443–478.

56. Szasz, T. (1988). *The Ethics of Psychoanalysis.* Syracuse, NY: Syracuse University Press, p. 53.

57. Kierkegaard, S. (1992). *Either/Or: A Fragment of a Life.* A. Hannay (Trans.). New York, NY: Penguin. (Original work published 1843); Kierkegaard, S. (2003). *Fear and Trembling.* A. Hannay (Trans.). New York, NY: Penguin. (Original work published 1843.)

58. Binswanger, L. (1963). *Being in the World: Selected Papers of Ludwig Binswanger.* J. Needleman (Trans.). New York, NY: Basic Books. (Original work published in 1942.)

59. Jaspers, K. (2014). *Existenzphilosophie.* Frankfurt: De Gruyter. (Original work published 1938.)

60. Yalom, I. (1980). *Existential Psychotherapy.* New York, NY: Basic Books.

61. Burston, D. (2000). R.D. Laing's contribution to existentialism and humanistic psychology. *Psychoanalytic Review,* 87(4): 549–560.

62. Atwood, G.E., Stolorow, R.D., & Orange, D.M. (2011). The madness and genius of post-Cartesian philosophy. *Psychoanalytic Review,* 98(3): 263–285.

63. Mills, J. (2003). Existentialism and psychoanalysis: from antiquity to post-modernism. *Psychoanalytic Review,* 90(3): 269–279.

64. Stolorow, R.D. (1997). Dynamic, dyadic, intersubjective systems: an evolving paradigm for psychoanalysis. *Psychoanalytic Psychology,* 14: 337–364; Stolorow, R.D. (2007). *Trauma and Human Existence: Autobiographical, Psychoanalytic, and Philosophical Reflections.* New York, NY: Analytic Press; Stolorow, R.D. (2008). The contextuality and existentiality of emotional trauma. *Psychoanalytic Dialogues,* 18(1): 113–123; Stolorow, R.D. (2011). *World, Affectivity, Trauma: Heidegger and Post-Cartesian Psychoanalysis.* New York, NY: Routledge; Stolorow, R.D. (2015). A phenomenological-contextual, existential, and ethical perspective on emotional trauma. *Psychoanalytic Review,* 102(1): 123–138; Stolorow, R.D. (2016). Using Heidegger. *Journal of the American Psychoanalytic Association,* 64: NP12–NP15.

65. Stolorow, R.D. (2008). The contextuality and existentiality of emotional trauma. *Psychoanalytic Dialogues,* 18(1): 113–123, p. 120.

66. Hoffman, I.Z. (2009). Doublethinking our way to "scientific" legitimacy: the desiccation of human experience. *Journal of the American Psychoanalytic Association,* 57(5): 1043–1069.

67. Houseman, A.E. (1994). *Collected Poems.* London: Wordsworth Editions.

68. Erikson, E. (1994). *Identity and the Life Cycle.* New York, NY: Norton.

69. Cocteau, J. (2013). *Opium: The Diary of his Cure.* M. Crosland (Trans.). London: Peter Owen.

CHAPTER 4

The evolution of psychoanalytic theory

On a blazing hot Southern California afternoon in the early 1990s, I drove Thomas Szasz from his hotel in Newport Beach to Pasadena. I had invited him to speak to a local psychoanalytic association in Pasadena, and he'd just finished another talk in Orange County. The traffic was terrible. The September afternoon glowed with the most perfect orange-reds of sunset, inviting us to settle into a lovely, long talk. If you know of him, you understand how tyrannical his writing seems. He shouts at you. Surprisingly, Szasz, in person, a small-statured man in his mid-seventies, behaved like a European gentleman. He spoke with gentle kindness. He revealed his passion only once, when slapping the dashboard with his hands to emphasize the non-medical nature of depth psychotherapy. When I shared my pride at my acceptance into a four-year, formal psychoanalytic training program, he quipped, "That will be good for you," adding, "but it need not take so long."

I remembered those words often while I attended weekly seminars, provided control cases (practice psychoanalyses conducted as part of the training process), attended weekly supervision sessions for each control case, and underwent a four-time-per-week training analysis.

Formal psychoanalytic training, particularly in America, parallels the medical school experience. Students in psychoanalytic training programs, especially the more formal, traditional ones, take an entire year of Freud—mirroring medical students spending their first year studying anatomy. I trained at the New Center for Psychoanalysis (NCP) in Los Angeles, which is accredited by the International and American Psychoanalytic Associations (IPA and APsaA). Though it leaned toward the conservative end, it nonetheless prided itself on its university style of education, exposing students to an array of psychoanalytic models from the classical to the contemporary. In the early 2000s, I passed written and oral examinations to achieve Certification in psychoanalysis, the gateway to anointment as a Supervising and Training Psychoanalyst. It was an absurd and traumatic experience. Senior psychoanalysts judged "objectively" what is, in truth, an extremely subjective process. They replied to written and oral descriptions of three of my control cases. In essence, they judged the beauty of a distorted art from a full continent away (because they interviewed me in New York, and I live in Los Angeles).

Psychoanalytic training involves studying the history and evolution of psychoanalytic theories of mind. Halfway through the process, the truth of Szasz' statement became obvious. Psychoanalytic training took too long. The clinical part should be an old-fashioned apprenticeship. It cannot be taught through books. Like any other type of art form—painting, writing, sculpting—learning depth psychotherapy requires extensive supervised practice. Students wishing to learn how to facilitate the transformational encounters ideally *do the work* with an experienced psychoanalyst, metaphorically, looking over their shoulder.

Depth psychotherapy requires primarily the capacity for improvisation,[1] for spontaneity, and for reactivity, and therefore interpersonal skills are most important. The training teaches you about the history of the field, i.e., how different psychoanalytic models of mind emerged and how they offer their own unique slant on how to promote personal transformation. Although I focus here primarily on explaining how actual psychoanalytic processes work, readers will benefit from a basic understanding of the history of psychoanalysis. I turn now to presenting such information even more quickly than Szasz counseled.

Parallels between intellectual and psychoanalytic history

The evolution of depth psychotherapy mirrors how other key ideas in intellectual history unfolded. These processes explain how psychoanalytic models of mind and practice have changed, and radically so, in the just more than a hundred-year history of the field. The history of the field begins, obviously, with the work of Sigmund Freud. A Caucasian Jewish man, Freud was the eldest of eight siblings. His family moved to Vienna when he was three. After completing a university degree, Freud studied medicine. He specialized in neurology. The antisemitism rampant in Austria prevented him from pursuing his preferred career of university teaching. Instead, he opened a private practice and continued studying on his own. As the nineteenth century transitioned into the twentieth, Freud received a scholarship to study with Jean-Martin Charcot[2] at the psychiatric hospital Salpêtrière in Paris. Charcot's use of hypnosis to stimulate pseudo-neurological symptoms, like seizures and fainting, captured Freud's attention. He was fascinated by hysterical phenomena, displayed by primarily female patients. He was intrigued by the intensity of the symptoms, which lacked any specific physiological basis.

Back in Vienna, Freud began treating such patients himself, first using hypnosis and later applying his own "talk therapy." It encouraged patients to remember traumatic events and the emotions associated with them. He collaborated with another physician, Josef Breuer, in developing the method. Together, they published their work with a patient, fictionally named Anna O.[3] She used the phrase "chimney sweeping" to describe the improvement she felt simply through the process of remembering and re-experiencing historically traumatic events. In an 1896 letter to his friend and physician, Wilhelm Fliess, Freud first coined the term, "psychoanalysis."[4] Thus, the new profession came into existence. Freud's subsequent writings formed long, winding tributaries. Other psychoanalysts of his era also began writing, creating their own tributaries, which joined into streams and, ultimately, into the ocean of psychoanalytic literature now in existence.

Scientism and empiricism dominated Freud's era. He sought an entirely rational, scientific basis for psychoanalysis, defining the field as "the science of unconscious mental processes."[5] However, the concept of the unconscious itself was hardly new. Ancient theologians and philosophers long understood how influences originating outside of consciousness affect behavior. They described how temptation, divine inspiration, and the gods unconsciously motivated people. Hinduism's central theological text, the Vedas, refers to unconscious aspects of mentality as early as two millennia BC. Without ever using the specific term, Shakespeare actively explores unconscious conflicts in his plays. The term, *unconscious*, was first introduced by the eighteenth-century German Romantic philosopher Friedrich Shelling. Coleridge first used the word in English. A panoply of Western philosophers, including Arthur Schopenhauer, Baruch Spinoza, Gottfried Leibniz, Johann Gottlieb Fichte, Georg Wilhelm Friedrich Hegel, Soren Kierkegaard, and Friedrich Nietzsche, referenced the unconscious in their work.

The unconscious remains the centerpiece of psychoanalysis. However, the concept of what constitutes the unconscious has evolved along with the rest of the Western intellectual tradition. Within a decade, Freud had identified three other phenomena as central to psychoanalytic work, and each related to the unconscious: the transference, the repetition compulsion, and dreams. As I discussed in the last chapter, the transference consists of a mapping of archaic, infantile relational patterns onto the psychoanalyst. In his 1914 paper "Remembering, repeating, and working through," Freud first introduced the concept:

> The patient does not *remember* anything of what he has forgotten and repressed, he *acts* it out, without, of course, knowing that he is repeating it ... For instance, the patient does not say that he remembers that he used to be defiant and critical toward his parents' authority; instead, he behaves that way to the doctor.[6]

Freud uses the transference to introduce the repetition compulsion, a phenomenon he expanded upon in his 1920 book, *Beyond the Pleasure Principle*. It is defined as the propensity to repeat traumatic or other self-destructive themes. Freud's original model of motivation, *Eros*, manifested as the pleasure principle. Attributing patients deliberately harming, or even killing themselves, to the pursuit of pleasure failed. It was for this reason that Freud introduced the concept of *Thanatos*, the death instinct. He knew it sounded oxymoronic, and he repeatedly mentions his struggle to find another way of explaining self-harming behaviors. The concept allowed him to expand his basic motivation for human behavior from the *Eros*, or seeking pleasure, to the dual-drive theory of *Eros* and *Thanatos*.

Arguably Freud's most important contribution, *The Interpretation of Dreams*, was published earlier, in 1900. In it, he proclaimed to have solved the puzzle of the meaning of dreams: They represent hidden wishes which seek fulfillment. A patient's dream of beating his father to death likely represents a hidden, unconscious wish to vanquish the father. Freud's work on dreams introduced four concepts relevant to interpreting the unconscious wherever uncovered: *symbolization*, *condensation*, *displacement*, and *secondary revision*.

Symbolization refers to the semiotic nature of dreaming. Your dream of your supervisor, an older male, for example, could represent him or her. However, it could equally stand for power, for masculinity, for authority, or an infinite number of related concepts. Condensation accounts for the possibility that the image can represent your father, grandfather, some other authority figure or *all* of those figures. Displacement refers to mental content moving around in dreams. Your dreaming of an argument with your romantic partner may well simply mimic your actual anger at him or her, but it may also, through displacement, represent the partner's anger at you or someone else's annoyance or irritation at you. Alternatively, the authority figure in the dream might represent you. Secondary revision describes the process through which we change dreams when we remember them. You might have *actually* dreamed that the supervisor murdered a coworker, but—because you would find the image disturbing—you remember it as a more benign injury. These are all unconscious processes. According to Freud, unconscious processes like displacement alter dreams to render them palatable. They allow us to continue sleeping.

Most psychoanalytic theorists offer differing versions of dream interpretation. They expand, reject, or edit Freud's original theory. I find Ronald Fairbairn's theory of dreams most compelling: They are short, abbreviated cinematic films representing unresolved conflicts, unmet need states, trauma, or other unsettled unconscious themes. It matters naught whether dreams are, as some assert, the result of random neurophysiological impulses. We create meaning out of them.

Freud's assertions that *dreamwork* consists of some type of encryption, of masking, or even, simply, of truncating these themes remain accurate. Interestingly, dreamwork mimics the mind's defense mechanisms— another concept accepted by psychoanalysts of various theoretical persuasions. Lacan famously considers the unconscious as structured like a language. He highlighted how metaphor, metonymy, and symbolization functions in language like defense mechanisms do in our minds.

Having introduced these three basic psychoanalytic concepts, Freud turned to considering how the mind was structured. He initially considered the unconscious as topographically ordered. Information passed from the unconscious to the preconscious and, finally, to consciousness, surmounting obstacles along the way. In 1923, with the publication of his *The Ego and the Id*, Freud introduced his tripartite theory. He designated the id as containing the reservoir of unstructured, powerful instinctual urges and drives, consisting of "a cauldron full of seething excitations."[7] Herein lie the drives, the realm where biological instincts meet the mental. They are powerful, disorganized, chaotic, and striving for satisfaction. Sexual, aggressive, and other primitive urges, and all of their derivatives, comprise the id. The superego is an unconscious structure consisting of internalized prohibitions and inhibitions derived from parental or societal influences. It directs the activities of the ego, guiding it according to moral or ethical strictures. The ego, the final arbiter between these two internal forces and external reality, forms the third part of Freud's structural model. He tweaked it in various ways up until his death, in London, in 1939.

The birth of object relations theories

Many of Freud's contributions, such as the idea that motivation is driven by two basic drives, remain in common usage. But the original Freudian model has morphed considerably. It has been expanded to include a desire for knowledge for knowledge's sake and a need for social connection that does not necessarily have sexuality as its basic component. Contemporary psychoanalysts like Joseph Lichtenberg[8] expand Freud's motivational model to include five basic motivations: needs to regulate physiological requirements like hunger or thirst, needs for attachment and affiliation, for exploration and assertion, abilities to react aversively through antagonism or withdrawal, and needs for sensual pleasure and sexual excitement.

Another of Freud's early papers, "Mourning and melancholia," contains the seeds of object relations theory. The theory proffers objectivist, scientific-sounding words, like objects, to describe the operations of the internal drama. It accounts for activities in the unconscious, inner world. However, theorists often use the word "object" to describe the impact of real persons in the interpersonal environment, creating unnecessary confusion. Freud believed melancholia, meaning clinical depression in contemporary language, results from an attack on the ego by an internal object. In essence, a part of the mind, identified with real persons like mother, father, or a conglomeration of childhood caregivers, attacks another part of the mind. It is one of psychoanalysis' first references to dynamic relationships developing between different parts of the ego.

Of course, concepts of the "internal drama" or inner life of persons appeared in literature, drama, and poetry for millennia prior to Freud. However, Freud's description of an internal ego-assault was a milestone in the field's history. Freud writes of how, in the state of melancholia, a relationship with such an external object is "transformed … into a cleavage between the critical activity of the ego and the ego as altered by identification."[9] He specifically identifies how identifications with outer critics create a "new agency" that carries on, internally, much like the formally external critics. The idea morphed into what he later called the superego.

Initial conceptions of the psychoanalyst–patient relationship

I learned the craft of depth psychotherapy well after the Freudian dominance of psychoanalysis declined. The timing was perfect because I could never practice the abstinence and neutrality required of the conservative Freudian disciples. In fact, I was mostly exposed to the modern, relationally oriented approaches to psychoanalysis. The scientism reigning supreme when Freud introduced the profession began waning. He had viewed the mind as a singular, independent entity. In his

1912 paper titled "Recommendations to physicians practicing psycho-analysis," Freud introduced psychoanalytic neutrality by writing:

> I cannot advise my colleagues too urgently to model them-selves during psycho-analytic treatment on the surgeon, who puts aside all his feelings, even his human sympathy, and con-centrates his mental forces on the single aim of performing the operation as skillfully as possible ... The justification for requir-ing this emotional coldness in the analyst is that it creates the most advantageous conditions for both parties: for the doctor a desirable protection for his own emotional life and for the patient the largest amount of help that we can give him to-day.[10]

Practitioners, Freud believed, wield a surgical-like objectivity. They interpret the unconscious in order to strengthen the ego. Using rea-son the same way as Socrates and Plato did centuries before him, Freud believed rationality could conquer the irrationality of the passions. In the *Republic*, Plato, Socrates' messenger and interpreter, suggested only prop-erly guided reason could conquer the appetites prone to enslave it. He and his student, Aristotle, considered reason the superior human qual-ity. Freud institutionalized their ancient wisdom, and packaged it into the purchasable service called psychoanalysis. The idea remained central to all subsequent psychoanalytic, psychodynamic, and other depth psy-chotherapeutic models of mind until the mid-twentieth century.

The original psychoanalytic relationship, then, was of an authoritarian nature, of expert to novice, of teacher to student, of master to slave. The psychodynamic psychotherapist's job consisted of interpreting the uncon-scious, particularly as it presented itself in the transference, the repeti-tion compulsion, and dreams. Like building muscles enhances a person's capacity for physical work, cognitive interpretations by psychoanalysts develop patients' ego capacity. The impact of the professional relationship itself figured little in the transformative process. In fact, Freud initially considered countertransference as pathological. He recommended practi-tioners undergo psychoanalysis every few years to, by analogy, keep their interpretive filter clean. He considered erotic feelings, aggression, or even benign emotions felt by psychoanalysts, whether stimulated by patients or arising within the practitioners themselves, irrelevant.

Sándor Ferenczi, who surprisingly remained within Freud's inner circle, was among the first of Freud's followers to question psychoanalytic neutrality. He worried practitioners unwittingly re-injured patients, particularly those subjected to childhood neglect. He recorded his ideas in his clinical diaries.[11] Ferenczi observed some of his patients reacting to his neutrality with hurt, describing some of them as calling him "insensitive, cold, even hard and cruel, [and] they reproached me with being selfish, heartless, conceited ..." These observations led him to the conclusion that "patients have an exceedingly refined sensitivity for the wishes, tendencies, whims, sympathies and antipathies of their analyst."[12] In other words, and speaking pure heresy, Ferenczi considered his patients' reactions to neutrality as real, and he also considered them as interested in *him*. Because these ideas severely countered Freud's fundamental rules of abstinence and neutrality, Ferenczi's ideas were marginalized until well after his death in 1933. They gained attention only as the intersubjective and relational approaches increased in popularity.

Although psychoanalysts began splintering into competing schools within the first decade of the field's existence, they retained their emphasis on one-person models. Jung considered context more broadly by, for example, introducing the collective unconscious with its universal archetypes.[13] Still, even Jungians emphasize one-person models of mind. Scattered references allude to interpersonal and intersubjective forces affecting individuals, but the emphasis remains on the unitary, individual mind. In effect, these early theorists focused on the psychodynamics of the individual-in-isolation.

Enter Ronald Fairbairn, the Scottish psychoanalyst whose theory developed in opposition to Melanie Klein's. Arguably the greatest split between the two theorists regards the origin of aggression emerging from *Thanatos*. In the simplest terms, Klein considered aggression an innate part of human nature—inescapable and unavoidable. Fairbairn thought it reactive. He argued that if a baby was only loved sufficiently, no need would exist for angry feelings to emerge. Although Klein thought a highly complex, internal drama was present at birth, Fairbairn believed the inner world only developed in reaction to depriving infantile experiences. Both Klein and Fairbairn most significantly laid the groundwork for the evolution of what Aron calls the "relational turn" in psychoanalysis.

Living and writing in Berlin, Budapest, and Vienna during the 1930s, the psychoanalysts of the era relocated to Britain after the rise of Nazism. They mostly fled to London, where they flourished in the liberal freedom of the country. They joined the British Psychoanalytic Institute. By the early 1940s, the Kleinians and the Freudians split from one another. These types of religious-like schisms litter the history of psychoanalysis. If you entered training in the British Psychoanalytic Institute during this period, you had to choose a school, either Freudian or Kleinian. Eventually, a third school also appeared, the middle, independent, or British object relations theorists. It is to those ideas I now turn, but only after expanding upon the foundations of them.

Klein's emphasis on the darkness of humanity

Klein's conceptualization of the internal drama was less tightly organized than Freud's. She and her followers focus on "unconscious phantasy."[14] They differentiate "fantasy," which is conscious, from "phantasy," which is unconscious. Regardless of how coherent, clear, or organized your conscious thought is, it arises from your unconscious fantasy life. While retaining the Freudian emphasis on instinctual drive, the Kleinian model delves deeper into the meaning-making function of the mind. The inner world is a battlefield, containing dramatic themes comparable to battles found in Homerian epics or Shakespearean plays.

According to the Kleinian model, infants begin life with weak and ill-defined self-images. Their minds are literally in pieces, full of fear, rage, envy, and similarly intense emotions. To reduce the emotional complexity of the world, they utilize a primitive defensive mechanism called splitting. Through an unconscious, possibly biologically based mechanism, they divide the world into categories of good and bad. The world of the infinite becomes reduced to the binary—a simpler, easier to manage, and ultimately anxiety-reducing view. This is called the qualitative split, with *schizoid* meaning splitting. When babies are fed, rested, and otherwise comfortable, the world is good. When conditions are uncomfortable, the world is bad. As infants mature, the simplifying function of splitting begins to falter.

Klein named this earliest phase of life, the one dominated by splitting first and projection second, as the "paranoid–schizoid" position.

She intentionally named it a position, instead of stage or phase, to denote how individuals never entirely mature out of this position. It persists in even the most mature individuals. The phrase accounts for the splitting processes noted above. The projection, in which badness or anger is perceived as in others, results in a primitive form of paranoia. In other words, infants' inner worlds are dominated by schizoid and paranoid experiences.

One of the more important, complex and confusing features of Klein's developmental theory concerns her use of the phrase, *projective identification*.[15] The term has since attracted lingering controversy. The simplest way to comprehend the phrase is to think of mental content as movable, like furniture in a room, within an individual's psyche, or even between different psyches. As I will demonstrate in greater detail soon, my personal feelings, like a loving parent to Carlos, or a rescuing caregiver to Gilda, or a frustrated colleague to Penn, all represent, in part, projective identifications. I was feeling *their* emotions, mixed in with my own. Emotional experiences, such as anger, can also be transferred between different parts of your own mind (known as intra-psychic projective identification). Anger, which may be unacceptable to experience consciously, could be transferred internally, strengthening the critical part. As a result, you might experience a sense of constant, internal oppression.

Projective identification may also be understood as a primitive form of communication. Consider the infant who cries out of hunger. Its mother often viscerally feels the infant's pain. This illustrates interpersonal projective identification. The infant's pain is somehow verbally and nonverbally transmitted to the mother in such a fashion that *she* feels it. As infants and toddlers evolve, projective identification gives way to more mature forms of communication. The common parental utterance to toddlers, "use your words," exemplifies efforts by parents to get children to convert projective identifications into language.

Kleinians believe that, somewhere between three and six months of age, babies begin to have serious problems as their images of self and other coalesce. Gradually, these all good or all bad images of self, or of other, become combined. Klein called the resulting crisis of integration the "depressive position," probably because of the inner conflict involved in realizing that you, and the person you love, contain both bad *and* good. Thus begins, then, the central moral problem of life: how to integrate loving and hating feelings. Other related but central moral and psychological issues follow from this. How can I take care of myself while still taking care of others? The depressive position accounts for the lifelong balancing act between excessive sacrifice, which leads to masochism, and insufficient sacrifice, which leads to narcissism. As the depressive position gains strength, primitive mechanisms, like splitting and projective identification, fall by the wayside. They are replaced by more mature defense mechanisms like repression, denial, sublimation, anticipation, and humor. These are all depressive position functions.

The paranoid–schizoid world does not recognize two or more people in a system. It is characterized by an infantile, highly narcissistic world-view in which the existence of the other is not subjectively realized. However poorly defined the sense of self might be, there is only one world: the world of the self. With the transition into the depressive position, the infant actually begins caring for others. Morality does not exist in the paranoid–schizoid position, and neither does empathy. Klein remained fairly close to the Freudian model of mind and practice. She believed in dual-drive theory, although she seemed, particularly in her early work, to emphasize the aggressive over the more loving aspects of these drives. She believed infants were born with innate anger and envy, which varied in intensity depending upon constitutional and/or early environmental factors. Klein softened her views in her later years, even entertaining some of the analyst–patient interplay privileged by more recent theories.[16] However, and for the most part, she remained devoted to the same Gemini twins of abstinence and neutrality.[17] She would hardly have considered the psychoanalytic relationship itself as curative.

Fairbairn's romantic vision

Fairbairn rejected Freud and Klein's biologically driven models. In contrast, he viewed the internal world as developing from entirely environmental factors, noting that: "psychopathological inquiry, which in the past has been successively focused, first upon impulse, and later upon the ego, [should] now be focused upon the object toward which the impulse is directed," adding that, "the time is now ripe for a psychology of object relationships ..."[18] The *crucial* ideological shift here—one *not* made by Klein or Freud—concerns Fairbairn's emphasis on the *social* nature of human persons. By implication, their internal dramas form from communal, social influences rather than from individualistic, instinct-driven ones.

While Freud, Klein, and their followers were busy elaborating on their individualized, hydraulic-like models of the mind, Fairbairn—in no small way a result of his working in relative isolation in Edinburgh—radically departed from them. He discarded the Freudian developmental stages of oral, anal, latent, and phallic. They represent instead, Fairbairn believed, the means through which infants attach to their mothers or caregivers. Fairbairn writes, "The ultimate goal of libido is the object; and in its search for the object libido is determined by similar laws to those which determine the flow of electrical energy, i.e., it seeks the path of least resistance."[19]

Fairbairn had studied philosophy, then Hellenic studies, and then theology. In the aftermath of World War I, he attended medical school and then trained in psychiatry. Like his predecessors, Fairbairn began as a Freudian, but then developed his own creative ideas. He was influenced by his work with schizoid patients—individuals who tend to withdraw into their own inner worlds. Fairbairn believed these individuals had been psychically damaged early in life, rendering their relationships with others tenuous. Unlike Freud or Klein, Fairbairn thought children were highly socially oriented from birth. They needed to be valued and enjoyed by their parents, not just have their instincts satisfied. For Fairbairn, anxiety originates in separation from the mother.

Fairbairn entirely discarded Freud's tripartite model. In its place, the psyche consisted primarily of an ego, or self, highly interactive from infancy. He believed the ego had its own energy without requiring fuel from the id. He considered libido as a sort of psychic electrical energy naturally oriented to connect to others. Our lungs breathe air, our eyes see light, our ears hear sounds, and our minds seek out other minds with which to interact. We are built that way; we cannot choose otherwise. Fairbairn was also the first theorist to indicate that aspects of self are always tied to aspects of other. He called these "dynamic structures."[20] For example, if you are enjoying this book, then part of your ego enjoys the experience, while some other part of the other, be it a representation of mother, father, or some other figure, is validating the experience. Fairbairn later developed a rather confusing model of how these internal dynamic structures relate to one another. Suffice to say that the psyche, as Phillip Bromberg would also attest, consists of a multiplicity of dynamic structures or a multiplicity of egos. We view the world through the lens of them.

Fairbairn also theorized that levels of psychopathology can be understood in terms of an infant's capacity to socially engage. Whether biologically or environmentally challenged, the infant who cannot attach well to caregiving figures will feel that its love is dangerous. Their primary conflict will be to love or not to love. If traumatized at this level, humans will withdraw into deeper schizoid states, and they may manifest in psychosis or borderline personality disorders. In brief, such children will feel as if their own love and need for connection is bad. They struggle with any kind of intimacy. If, in contrast, a child feels that their love is accepted, then their conflict correspondingly becomes one of whether to suck or to bite, or to love or to hate. Note the similarity to the Kleinian idea of the depressive position. These individuals primarily fear the loss of the object or the other.

Fairbairn did not believe in the superego in the Freudian sense. He thought, instead, that the unconscious consists of a considerable amount of self-hatred because, again, the child has internalized negative images of self in order to keep the external world good. He called this the moral defense. Listen for the influence of his theological training in these excerpts from his writing. Regarding the need to keep others on the outside, such as parental figures, good and strong, and speaking to the universal struggle with self-esteem with which we all struggle, Fairbairn writes:

> To say that the child takes upon himself the burden of badness which appears to reside in his objects is, of course, the same thing as to say that he internalizes his bad objects. The sense of outer security resulting from this process of internalization is, however, liable to be seriously compromised by the resulting presence within him of internalized bad objects. Outer security is thus purchased at the price of inner insecurity; and his ego is henceforth left at the mercy of a band of internal fifth columnists or persecutors, against which defenses have to be, first hastily erected, and later laboriously consolidated.[21]

Fairbairn's model leaves little room for innate, biological factors, ushering in the more contemporary, relational psychoanalytic schools. Infant observational studies confirm that some babies are better at attaching to mothers than others, regardless of the competency of the parental figures involved. In all likelihood, the internal world is a combination of some *a priori* images, as suggested by Klein, which are then shaped and formed by environmental factors, as suggested by Fairbairn.

Other middle school contributions

While not attaining the same fame as the other middle school theorists, several other scholars made important contributions to this mid-twentieth-century change. Donald Winnicott, pediatrician turned psychoanalyst, introduced several key ideas. He, like many middle school theorists, never introduced a comprehensive theory of mind as had Freud, Jung, Klein, and Fairbairn. For example, Winnicott introduced the concept of primary maternal preoccupation—a phenomenon in which a mother becomes highly preoccupied with her baby several months before it is born and then around a year afterwards. The love and attention showered on the child builds a strong, competent sense of self. When caregivers are out of tune with their charges, babies develop what Winnicott called the false self.[22] They assess what their parents need, and alter their behaviors to please them. Their true self goes into hiding. In the same spirit, Winnicott famously proclaimed that mothers and babies do not exist; only mother–infant units do.

Michael Balint introduced the concept of the basic fault,[23] namely a vulnerability within an individual's personality that causes splits and disintegration to occur from that point forward. He writes,

> In my view the origin of the basic fault may be traced back to a considerable discrepancy in the early formative phases of the individual between his biopsychosocial needs and the material and psychological care, attention, and affection available during the relevant times. This creates a state of deficiency whose consequences and after-affects appear to be only partly reversible.[24]

Balint used the word "fault" because many of his patients literally used that word. They told him they had a fault within them that needed correction. Balint believed these fault lines resulted from mis-attunements by parents or other caregivers, and later manifested in psychoanalytic relationships "as a desperate demand, but this time the analyst should not—in fact must not—fail him."[25] Balint posited the presence of what he called primary love, a type of interpenetrating immersion of love between parent and child. Such an intense bond helps to create a healthy sense of self—a concept paralleling Winnicott's concept of caregiver–infant as a fused unit as well as his concept of primary maternal preoccupation. For Balint, the provision of a sufficient amount of primary love minimizes or prevents the development of the basic fault. He thought depth psychotherapists regressed patients back to where the basic fault was, and helped them to progress from there. Thus, the origin of another of his phrases, "regression for the sake of progression."[26]

More recently, Thomas Ogden offers several additional concepts relevant to these middle object relations theorists. He criticizes Klein's model because of its reliance upon unstructured unconscious fantasies; he criticizes Freud for failing to place energy in the ego. Most significantly, he updated Fairbairn's concept of "dynamic structures" by coining the phrase "ego suborganizations"[27] to describe how "internal objects [could become] heavily identified with an object representation while maintaining the capacities of the whole ego for thought, perception, feeling, etc."[28] Here, Odgen helpfully explains how internal dramas become dynamic, complex, and conflict-ridden. By identifying the internal drama as a form of imprinting on the ego itself, Ogden accounted for the dynamism eluding Fairbairn and Klein's more static descriptions of the inner world. Also, he introduced the idea of the "analytic third,"[29] emphasizing the effect of the analytic relationship on both parties and moving the profession toward greater consideration of interpersonal features. Contemporary object relational theorists such as Christopher Bollas, James Grotstein, and Bromberg further elucidated this model, also viewing the unconscious as populated by variations of internal dramas.

The late twentieth-century transition in psychoanalysis

These middle school object relations theories ushered in a major paradigm shift later in the twentieth century. Within two decades, Klein, Fairbairn, and the subsequent object relations theorists laid the groundwork for the development of these more interpersonal models of mind. As so often occurs in the history of any field, ideas became clustered into categories. In London, which became the center of psychoanalysis after the 1930s, three schools existed: Those still adhering to traditional psychoanalysis, led by the field's heir apparent, Sigmund Freud's daughter, Anna Freud; those following Klein; and the British object relations school, which included Donald Winnicott, Wilfred Bion, Michael Balint, Jay Sutherland, John Bowlby, and others. Many consider that a major revision of psychoanalysis evolved from this latter paradigm, one privileging the developing mother–infant relationship and viewed as the metaphorical foundation of the actual psychoanalytic relationship.

The idea of psychoanalytic relationships having a mutative, curative function only entered the mainstream of psychoanalytic thinking as the sociopolitical landscape changed. Elisabeth Young-Bruehl[30] believes that a synthesis of social progressivism emerging from the ashes of World War II facilitated this change in psychoanalysis. The devastations, losses, abandonments, and traumatic experiences of that war led to a greater emphasis on the emotional needs of vulnerable children and adults, paving the way for psychoanalysts to highlight the "basic human drive for attachment and security."[31] Later in the twentieth century, the burgeoning controversy regarding the precise aims of psychoanalysis flowed into two increasingly turbulent streams. Many psychoanalytic practitioners remained devoted to the exclusively medical vision. They applied various techniques such as confronting ego defenses—thereby exposing and resolving the painful unconscious conflicts or deficits they were masking. Using the *sine qua non* of the psychoanalytic process, these analysts focused on transference as the vehicle for the transformational process. They relied on the scientific method for gaining greater understanding of psychoanalysis. In meetings they would call "scientific," these psychoanalysts shared their findings, described their cases, and expanded their knowledge. In the present day, psychoanalysts of this ilk eagerly await advances in the neurosciences, conduct observational studies of infants, and immerse themselves in cognitive psychology research, hoping to establish a logical-positivistic basis for psychoanalysis. They believe the field will persist as one weapon among many, alongside psychopharmacology and cognitive behavioral therapy, in the battle against mental illness.

Other psychoanalysts applied their techniques with broader strokes. They utilized their training to help those with difficulties defying traditional medical categorization, such as persons who felt alienated, failed to enjoy romantic intimacies, felt inadequate, or found their life meaningless. These analysts eschewed the medical, scientific approach. They viewed their work as more of a hermeneutical, exploratory process than one solely intended to cure illnesses. They read outside of their field—literature, philosophy, and history—seeking support in these realms of knowledge. They viewed these disciplines as offering more meaningful insights into human subjectivity than could be garnered from the sciences.

Kohut's destruction of ego psychology

Breaking the yoke of the ego psychology which dominated psychoanalysis since it came to the US during the 1920s, Heinz Kohut[32] fractured the original Freudian psychoanalytic paradigm (much like Fairbairn had done previously). He spent most of his career as an avid follower of original Freudian thought. However, mostly resulting from his work with narcissistic patients, Kohut thought deficits deserved as much attention as conflicts. In essence, what patients missed in their childhoods—attention, curiosity, love—needs repair. Freud had considered these primitively injured patients inaccessible to psychoanalytic methods. Kohut disagreed, and like Fairbairn had a few decades earlier, introduced an entirely new model. Resulting in greater popularity because it deviated from the American psychoanalytic tradition so dramatically, Kohut introduced the idea of the cohesive self in place of Freud's ego, id, and superego. Self-psychology entered the fray, a school of its own.

Like Freud, Kohut championed a talking cure, striving to understand individuals within their subjective experiences by facilitating introspection. Also, like Freud, he utilized interpretation as a vehicle for change. While retaining an essentially one-person model, Kohut moved psychoanalysis deeper into the interpersonal realm. Psychoanalysts offer what he called a self-object function, a type of empathy or presence. Such attention facilitated the development of the cohesive self. In self-psychology, Kohut highlights empathy as the tool *par excellence*, allowing a relationship to develop between psychoanalysts and patients that offers some hope of mitigating early pathology in the development of the self.

Here, the ubiquity of overlap between ideas from various psychoanalysts, from Freud onward, becomes evident. Kohut's nomenclature differs significantly from Fairbairn's, but it is, in many ways, a similar model. You take away an empathic embrace of the child, what Winnicott refers to as the "holding environment,"[33] and the child is injured. Kohut equivocated regarding the curative capacity of psychoanalytic relationships. On the one hand, he introduced the concept of a "transmuting internalization,"[34] directly suggesting patients ingest their psychoanalysts, or the relationship itself, in a transformative manner; on the other hand, he warned psychoanalysts to beware of any omnipotent fantasies of believing they can fully re-parent their patients.

Kohut's model of development is fairly straightforward. Assuming intact neurobiology, infants, toddlers, and children require the type of external attention noted above to create *self-objects*. These are what the object relations theorists would have called caring or soothing internal objects. Kohut gives them a specific name, and emphasizes their role in psychological development. What more biologically oriented theorists would have termed "weaning," Kohut believed consisted of parents gradually (and unconsciously) transferring self-object functioning into their children. They must experience separation, frustration, and other painful developmental experiences to pave the way for development of the cohesive self.

Whereas the Freudian model featured a horizontal split in which repression works like a force field to keep unwanted material, unfiltered drives and urges, and other bothersome components out of consciousness, Kohut's model features a vertical one. The psyche consists of self-states or different fragments of self. The greater the psychopathology, the larger the spaces between the self-states. The extreme narcissism displayed by Carlos, as well as the psychogenic fugue states Gilda developed, are easily explained by Kohut's model. Carlos' grandiose, narcissistic self serves as a shield, a self-state protecting his underlying emotional vulnerability. In the midst of one of the hypnotic-like spells, Gilda's personality became overshadowed by one particular self-state. Her other ones went unconscious, silent.

If they lack sufficient emotional support during development, children develop fractures in the cohesiveness of the self. Narcissistic personality features, the fulcrum for Kohut's model, result from a person unconsciously installing an overly idealized, grandiose sense of self to compensate for deep insecurity. The degree of the split between the self and the idealization causes the psychopathology. Individuals with extreme narcissistic defenses are highly sensitive to even minor slights, let alone overt rejections. Variations in psychopathology may be conceptualized in a like manner. The psychotic person suffers from severe splits in self; the compulsive over-worker likely relies upon work to serve a self-object function because of a deficit in their own internal world.

Revolving around the concept of the self-object function, practitioners of self-psychology view the transference in unique ways. They accept, and expect, an idealizing transference to develop as patients re-experience their need for an omnipotent, adoring parental figure. Another variation is the twinship transference in which psychoanalyst and patient are both viewed in idealistic terms. My early work with Carlos clearly represents this type of transference. He was perfect; I was perfect; we were perfect. Kohut also called this the alter-ego transference. He believes transference unfolds like normal developmental processes—an archaic merger reflecting the primitive infant–caregiver relationship, the alter-ego transference or twinship, and the less archaic form of the mirror transference. The latter, for example, occurs with more mature patients.

Coming from a scientific, medical background, Kohut retained the use of empirical-sounding phrases like the "approving-mirroring functions of an admiring self-object."[35] These describe the way infants respond to parental attention, patients respond to their psychodynamic psychotherapist's attunement, and people feel, internally, the glow of their own positive self-regard. He leaped past psychoanalysts like Alexander with his corrective emotional experience. Kohut thought psychoanalysis works by facilitating patients' internalization of the self-object function of practitioners. These result in more positive self-images as well as more cohesive selves. One of his followers, John Lindon, used the phrase "optimal provision"[36] to describe how psychoanalysts' use of actual caring for patients facilitated the transformational process. Here, then, the radical suggestion, made by the pediatrician Winnicott, becomes concretized. Patients improve, at least in part, because their psychoanalytic sessions provide them with a form of re-parenting.

You would think a clinician like Kohut, with such a caring stance, would have ventured further in exploring the field between caregivers and infants, or between psychoanalysts and patients. He did not. He writes, "With psychoanalysis man has succeeded in transforming intro-spection and empathy into the tools of an empirical science."[37] Here, and again, Kohut betrays a lingering devotion to positivism, insisting as he does on utilizing empathy as a scientific tool. His choice of words and terms—modernist and objectivist in tone and consonant with his own time in history and culture—betray his persistent adherence to a one-person psychology.

In addition to alienating himself from his fellow ego psychologists and other adherents to the more conservative, Freudian models, Kohut's work drew criticism from other circles. Otto Kernberg, for example, vehemently disagrees with Kohut's marginalizing of the phenomenon of negative transference or of aggression in general. If working with the same narcissistic patient, Kernberg might aggressively confront the patient with the archaic nature of their defenses. Kohut would behave in a diametrically opposite manner, carefully listening and offering empa-thy rather than confrontations. Psychoanalysts who privilege drive theory would, in general, take issue with self-psychology. Followers of Lacan, who continue in the Freudian tradition with highly cognitive, language-based analyses, would view the self-psychologists as caught up in their *own* narcissism. They disagree that empathy is even possible, suggesting it emerges only after filtering through the mind of psychoan-alysts. It is thereby contaminated. Object relation theorists likely object to the simplicity of Kohut's model. In place of the dynamic structures hypothesized by Fairbairn, for example, self-psychologists see only fractured selves and inadequate self-objects. No place exists, they might argue, for the type of conflicted internal dramas most of us experience.

Intersubjectivity enters the scene

Arguably validating Freud's Oedipus complex, one of Kohut's early followers, Robert Stolorow, created the field of intersubjectivity dur-ing the 1980s. He studied originally with H.A. Murray[38] at Harvard, a proponent of personology. Later, he trained in Kohut's model, becoming intrigued by the contexts involved in psychoanalyst–patient interactions. Stolorow, with a keen-enough interest in philosophy to drive him to pursue a doctorate in it, along with his close associate, George Atwood, grounded themselves in Kohut's doctrines. Reflecting on how the personalities of psychoanalytic scholars shaped their models, the two scholars published *Structures of Subjectivity: Explorations in Psychoanalytic Phenomenology*.[39] Subsequent books and articles by the two men, as well as by like-minded scholars like Jessica Benjamin and Donna Orange, delved into the complexity of psychoanalytic relationships. They ultimately considered the entire phenomenon of mind to be contextually based, discarding all prior one-person models. Sounding a bit like self-psychologists, Stolorow and Atwood propose that the unconscious is *not* comprised of "repressed instinctual drive derivatives, but of affect states that have been defensively walled off because they failed to evoke attuned responsiveness from the early surround."[40] Later, Stolorow strayed even more so from instincts, toward a phenomenological contextualism with a central focus on dynamic intersubjective systems. Stolorow's model of phenomenological contextualism considers any conceptualization of the individual mind as erroneous, a remnant of Cartesian thinking. He fully embraces the interactivity of internal and external worlds, noting how,

> Recurring patterns of intersubjective transaction within the developmental system give rise to principles (thematic patterns, meaning-structures, cognitive-affective schemas) that unconsciously organize subsequent emotional and relational experiences.[41]

In the decades after the mid-twentieth century, and as time slid toward the 21st century, numerous psychoanalysts ventured out into that mysterious interpersonal and intersubjective field.

In fairness, many object relations theorists had previously described how subtle interpersonal influences pass both ways in psychoanalytic relationships. Ogden introduced the idea of the "analytic third," meaning unique properties of the two parties infusing their relationship. The evolution from the intrapsychic to the intersubjective views of transference began with Klein's introduction of the concept of projective identification, and then continued with Bion's container–contained formulation. The Barangers considered the analytic field as ripe for receiving, and enacting, patients' primitive fantasies. Indeed, with their introduction of the concept of the "bi-personal field,"[42] these theorists also traveled into how interpersonal influences affect patient and psychoanalyst, and how they shape our human experiences in general.

Psychoanalysis became viewed as an interplay between the two psyches existing in the consulting room, always affected by other contextual factors—the weather, the amount of oxygen in the air, nutritional factors, current events, and so on. Transference and countertransference also became viewed more broadly, as more of a totality of the feelings and reactions that the two parties experience toward each other. The transition away from one-person psychology progressed. Stolorow, his colleagues, and many theorists who followed him, remained steadfast in refusing to consider concepts of mind as reducible to individual structures like a cohesive self or a multiplicity of egos. Instead, mind exists *always* within contexts—interpersonal, sociocultural, biological, and so on *ad infinitum*. The static conception of self emerges, as the Buddhists preach, only as colored by contextual factors. Neither transference nor countertransference survive in the same manner they were previously viewed.

Other field theories

While not direct adherents to intersubjectivity theory, other psychoanalysts ventured into the murky realm of the field between persons. Robert Galatzer-Levy, for example, integrates concepts from quantum mechanics, relativity, and chaos theory to propose a radical revision of psychoanalytic theorizing. He believes chaos theory accounts for the complexities of natural, real systems—like unfolding psychoanalytic processes—better than classical physics, calling it "a promising candidate for a different form of theorizing than has previously been used in psychoanalysis."[43] Given the complexity of biology, particularly interacting with social, cultural, and historical dynamic themes, aggression remains of great interest to psychoanalysis, but, and again, it cannot be reduced to a hypothetical, one-person psychological construct. Anger, for example, cannot be considered to result from pent-up aggressive urges, the death instinct, a frustrated anti-libidinal ego, or a dissociated sense of self.

The way I tend to think of it, you can look at mental phenomena from any number of angles, but you cannot freeze them in place. Certainly, people have personality traits; they often develop rigid ways of dealing with trauma endured during their early childhood or later in their lives. However, these trends *always* exist in a context. They constantly evolve and change over time. This conclusion leads more credence to the idea, shared by Greenberg and Wallerstein, that psychoanalytic theory offers useful metaphors. A patient fascinated by mythology who studies cultural anthropology and remembers her dreams will likely present material for which Jungian metaphors prove most useful; in a like manner, the more primitive patient, filled with envious rage and relying primarily upon projective identification, will likely respond best to metaphors from Kleinian models.

Relational psychoanalysis

The roots of the third recent trend in psychoanalytic theorizing, relational psychoanalysis, are difficult to discern. Most credit Stephen Mitchell, a New York psychoanalyst who died suddenly and prematurely in the year 2000, at age fifty-four, with introducing the term. However, Mitchell himself believed the model resulted from combining the interpersonal emphasis of Harry Stack Sullivan—a psychiatrist who was not a psychoanalyst—with various object relations theories. Other theorists offering ideas consistent with the relational models include Sándor Ferenczi and Sabina Spielrein—both practitioners working in the field within the first few decades of its inception. Contemporary adherents include Aron, Emmanuel Ghent, Adrienne Harris, Nancy Chodorow, Irwin Z. Hoffman, Owen Renik, and Jessica Benjamin, the latter particularly known for introducing feminism into the psychoanalytic mainstream. The Boston Change Process Study Group addresses microstructures of psychoanalytic interaction to study vicissitudes in the way that the transference relationship unfolds over time.

The book, *Object Relations in Psychoanalytic Theory*,[44] authored by Stephen Mitchell and Jay Greenberg, summarized the history of psychoanalytic theory up to and including the introduction of the relational models. The book has proved, to date, one of the best-selling books in the field. The two men helpfully created two simple categories for the psychoanalytic models. There were the "drive-structural"[45] ones, represented by Freud's, Klein's, and even Fairbairn's models as I described earlier. The second category of "relational-structural"[46] approaches consists of models of mind emphasizing the role of two parties, and greater contextual factors, in creating the types of organizing themes to which Stolorow refers.

It remains difficult to differentiate relational psychoanalysis from intersubjectivity theory. Adherents insist on significant differences. Relational psychoanalysis invites practitioners to be more authentic, real others in patients' lives. The intersubjectivists, in contrast, almost lean toward one-person psychologies. They may utilize the contextual factors in their thinking about patients, but respond with more interpretations than self-disclosures. Relational psychoanalysis emphasizes the real-time presentation of internal dynamics within the psychoanalytic relationship, not so much in terms of the context of an individual but in terms of how it possesses the psychoanalytic relationship itself. Relational psychoanalysis also distinguishes itself by emphasizing the effect of real interpersonal relationships on development. Therefore, it essentially ignores traditional drive theory. Relationalists argue that relating with others is humans' *primary* motivation. Experiences with caregivers during early childhood significantly shape people's lives, but so do contemporary relationships. Therein lies their explanation of the repetition compulsion. Rather than a desire to master a traumatic situation, these interpersonal patterns repeat themselves because they mirror their infantile, archaic ones.

Relational psychotherapists have no qualms about entering a *real* relationship with their patients, and they privilege authenticity. They liberally self-disclose. They loathe separating transference out from the *actual* professional relationship. They conceive transference and countertransference as features of *all* relationships. Whereas a more traditional psychoanalyst might interpret transference as a function of projection, the relationalist would consider the relationship as immersed in it. No wonder student clinicians struggle to distinguish the intersubjective models from the relational ones. Indeed, the boundaries between these approaches seem fluid. Both models fully embrace the mid-twentieth-century shift, embracing Winnicott's holding environment and similar metaphors capturing how patients internalize their psychoanalysts and the psychoanalytic relationship. Critics believe relational psychoanalysis marginalizes the unconscious, but no evidence supports the critique. Perhaps the most reliable difference concerns the nature of the professional relationship itself. As noted, intersubjectivists manifest more one-person thinking, using interpersonal and other contextual factors in forming their interventions; relationalists work almost entirely into the two-person model. They destroy what Stolorow calls the myth of the individual mind, always privileging what occurs in the psychoanalytic relationship. The relationship itself can address deficits as well as conflicts, and can, in and of itself, provide a healing experience. Ideally, even liberal relational psychoanalysts eschew the "rent-a-friend" practiced by some lesser experienced psychotherapists. However, the professional relationship might look much like just that— an intense, asymmetrically intimate relationship which is scrutinized by the co-participants for unconscious material, transference manifestations, repetitive themes, and the other endless manifestations of the unconscious.

The contemporary scene

Strong adherents to classical Freudian, Kleinian, and similar models (like Lacan's) continue to practice depth psychotherapy around the globe. Strangely, they are distributed unequally. South America, for some reason, has an unusual proportion of Kleinian psychoanalysts. A few hard-core Freudians can still be found in the dark cavernous buildings of mid-town Manhattan. Paralleling the trendiness of major cosmopolitan areas, the more recent psychoanalytic schools, specifically self-psychology, intersubjectivity, and relational psychoanalysis, tend to thrive mostly in major metropolitan areas like Los Angeles, London, and New York. Heinz Kohut proudly hails from Chicago, and a number of self-psychology practitioners continue to work in the area.

Meanwhile, after more than a hundred years of splintering and fracturing, the disintegration continues. Why? A half-century ago, George Klein (1976)[47] considered any psychoanalytic theory of mind flawed because it impossibly intended to create objectivity from subjectivity. Stolorow ultimately concluded, that identifying static, psychoanalytic theories of mind may prove forever elusive. He heralded clinical psychoanalysis for its search for disavowed intentionality and unconscious meanings from the patient's experiences. However, he considered psychoanalysis' search for a theory of mind futile. Szasz reached a similar conclusion years earlier, observing that psychoanalysts

> differ from medical specialists who are experts in a particular group of diseases (e.g., the dermatologist or ophthalmologist), but resemble those who are experts in a particular technique (e.g., the roentgenologist [radiologist] or surgeon).[48]

Essentially, psychodynamic psychotherapists practice a specific type of transformation. They are best served by staying with the treatment, and avoiding static theories of mind. Recently, Stolorow and Atwood reached a similar conclusion, viewing psychoanalysis as, ideally, a form of phenomenological inquiry purged of metapsychological contaminants. In brief, consider using psychoanalytic metaphors as roughly hewn maps of the geography. And remember that, like actual maps, they always fall short of the actual terrain. Moreover, even recent findings in neurophysiology establish the uniqueness of each individual brain, even between identical twins. Persons are therefore incredibly unique, rendering limited any map of them.

The psyche–soma, to use one of Winnicott's neologisms, exists as a verb, not a noun. Any effort to concretize it, whether in terms of drives, emotions, or structures like ego, id, or superego, fails because of our dynamic existence. Humans constantly move. They literally move through space. They develop over time. Three millennia of philosophy and theology failed to deliver universals of human nature. Why should the depth psychotherapies fare any better? The four categories of phenomena of consistent interest to psychoanalysts—the unconscious, transference, the repetition compulsion, and dreams (and other signs of the unconscious mind)—survive the test of time. However, they, too, differ in terms of presentation, depending on the patient, and in the terms used to describe them, and on the particular psychoanalyst.

Although systematization exists through the four tenets now repeatedly mentioned, no actual technical interventions are possible, nor is the privileging of any specific theory. Greenberg and Mitchell view the application of psychoanalytic theory as "a matter of personal choice."[49] I would argue against their free-flowing proclamation by suggesting, instead, that it should be the choice of each psychoanalytic dyad. It is easy to find, whether reviewing ego psychology or archetype psychology, the four central tenets of psychoanalysis. What matters is what applies, what can be constructed, to use Hoffman's term, between psychoanalysts and their patients.[50]

Contemporary intersubjective, self-psychology, and relational psychoanalysts perform their work, struggling with the asymmetrical closeness necessary for transformation, no longer burdened with the mandate that they behave like surgeons. Instead, they behave more like lovers, as Renik (1993) implies when he proclaims, "effective clinical psychoanalysis is not unlike good sex."[51] They create a containing, holding, protective environment, staying attuned to their patients and providing them with high levels of close, careful listening and attention. They embrace Winnicott's oft-quoted phrase that it is "a joy to be hidden, but a disaster not to be found."[52]

The myriad models just reviewed validate the natural human striving to capture human psychology, to categorize it. Except for the true believers, most psychoanalytic psychotherapists select models from the psychoanalytic opus that best suit a particular patient at a particular moment in time. Highly competitive young men struggling with their fathers bring Freud's drive theory and his use of the Oedipus complex to mind. Patients who immerse themselves in mythology, seek out the themes in theater and cinema, and remember many of their dreams invite Jungian metaphors. Those reporting strong levels of envy and aggressiveness elicit ideas from Melanie Klein's work. As Atwood and Stolorow confirmed, psychoanalysts tended to form theoretical models based on their own personalities. I would add that the particular population with whom they worked, as well as their time in history, also shaped their thinking. Nonetheless, the models depth psychotherapists developed, and continue to develop, offer useful tools for practitioners and patients alike. They allow patients a cognitive framework, a language for understanding themselves and others.

In other words, we psychodynamic therapists would be well served by embracing the foundation of mystery I presented in the last chapter. Patients enter consulting rooms, report whatever concerns them, and they then proceed, in partner-like fashion with their psychoanalysts, to unravel the mystery of their subjectivities and their relationships. Dynamic trends and themes can certainly be identified; however, the type of scientific certitude sought by Freud and his colleagues in the early years of the field remains impossible. If you pursue any mental phenomenon, a persistent sense of sadness, for example, the causative factors are literally infinite. The complexity of the central nervous system as it interacts with social, cultural, and historical themes renders understanding the source of the sadness literally impossible. Part of the beauty of depth psychological work is that the search itself, for meanings and causes of emotional states like sadness, typically helps patients. The two parties, overpowered by the humbling dynamism of the factors affecting both practitioner and patient, find a way forward. In any event, and as this review of psychoanalytic models validates, the parties to depth psychotherapy need not submit to the complexity of mental phenomena in the sense of feeling diminished by it. They *must*, however, surrender to the impossibility of achieving a full, categorical understanding. Interestingly, psychoanalytic processes consist of a type of structured conversation, an exploration of the mind. It is the exploration itself, the partnership, that ultimately creates change. It is not finding certitude.

In the final analysis, and harkening back to the philosophical foundations presented, it is time we psychoanalysts relinquish our search for ineffable truth. Instead, and armed with our capacities for managing transformative relationships, we seek organizing trends, a function of the *Critic*, while framing the relationship and caring for the patient, a function of the *Lover*. All patients' dramatic internal worlds are nested in deeper themes. Neurobiology, for example, can of course greatly shape the form that our internal dynamic world takes. Cultural anthropology provides yet another nesting function. None of our internal worlds have been the same since 9/11. When I hear a loud bang in my Pasadena office, I look out my window to see if a mushroom cloud is blossoming over downtown Los Angeles. This type of internal persecutory expectation was created by a cultural event, not by maternal deprivation, biology, or any other phenomena.

The more recent emphasis on intimacy in psychoanalytic relation-ships requires psychoanalysts to exercise caution in how they provide their unique transformational services. They remain responsible for maintaining the frame. They sell a service—better-called sets of *trans-formational encounters* rather than psychotherapy—and must do so in a fashion that honors the integrity of their work and, of course, their patients. The person of the patient matters the most. In searching for that authentic being, the psychoanalytic process must be as open and free-flowing as possible. William Baranger writes:

> When all is said and done, the analytic process that is about to take place between analyst Z and analysand A is completely unforesee-able. It implies on the part of the analyst a perspective, more or less exact, more or less mistaken, that may—or may not—be modifi-able, depending on the circumstances, during the actual process. The process is a personal matter all through its unfolding.[53]

Free-flowing, yes, but depth psychotherapists must nonetheless main-tain certain limits and boundaries, which, yes, is the topic of the next chapter.

Notes

1. Ringstrom, P. (2001). Cultivating the improvisational in psychoanalytic treat-ment. *Psychoanalytic Dialogues*, 11: 727–754.
2. Charcot, J.M. (1889). *Clinical Lectures on Diseases of the Nervous System. [Leçons sur les maladies du système nerveux].* T. Savill (Trans.). London: The New Sydenham Society. (Original work published in 1878.)
3. Freud, S. (1895). *Studies on Hysteria. The Standard Edition of the Complete Psychological Works of Sigmund Freud, Volume II (1893–1895): Studies on Hysteria.* London: Hogarth Press, pp. 253–305.
4. Gay, P. (1988). *Freud: A Life for our Time.* New York, NY: Norton, p. 103.
5. Freud, S. (1925). *An Autobiographical Study. The Standard Edition of the Com-plete Psychological Works of Sigmund Freud, Volume XX.* London: Hogarth Press, pp. 1–76.
6. Freud, S. (1914). Remembering, repeating and working-through (further recommendations on the technique of psycho-analysis II). *The Standard*

Edition of the Complete Psychological Works of Sigmund Freud, Volume XII (1911–1913): The Case of Schreber, Papers on Technique and Other Works. London: Hogarth Press, pp. 145–156.

7. Freud, S. (1933). *New Introductory Lectures on Psycho-Analysis. The Standard Edition of the Complete Psychological Works of Sigmund Freud, Volume XXII (1932–1936): New Introductory Lectures on Psycho-Analysis and Other Works.* London: Hogarth Press, pp. 1–182.

8. Lichtenberg, J.D. (1989). *Psychoanalysis and Motivation.* Hillsdale, NJ: The Analytic Press.

9. Freud, S. (1917). Mourning and melancholia. *The Standard Edition of the Complete Psychological Works of Sigmund Freud, Volume XIV (1914–1916): On the History of the Psycho-Analytic Movement, Papers on Metapsychology and Other Works.* London: Hogarth Press, pp. 237–258.

10. Freud, S. (1912). Recommendations to physicians practicing psycho-analysis. *The Standard Edition of the Complete Psychological Works of Sigmund Freud, Volume XII (1911–1913): The Case of Schreber, Papers on Technique and Other Works.* London: Hogarth Press, pp. 109–120.

11. Ferenczi, S. (1995). *The Clinical Diary.* Cambridge, MA: The Harvard University Press.

12. Ferenczi, S. (1949). Confusion of the tongues between the adults and the child (the language of tenderness and of passion). *International Journal of Psychoanalysis*, 30: 225–230, p. 225.

13. Jung, C.G. (1972). *Two Essays on Analytic Psychology.* R.F.C. Hull (Trans.). Princeton, NJ: Princeton University Press.

14. Klein, M. (1946). Notes on some schizoid mechanisms. *The International Journal of Psychoanalysis*, 27: 99–110.

15. Ibid.

16. Klein, M. (1975). Envy and gratitude and other works 1946–1963. *International Psychoanalytic Library*, 104: 1–346. London: The Hogarth Press and the Institute of Psycho-Analysis.

17. Davies, J.M. (1994). Love in the afternoon: a relational reconsideration of desire and dread in the countertransference. *Psychoanalytic Dialogue*, 4: 153–170. Doi: 10.1080/10481889409539011.

18. Fairbairn, W.R.D. (1952). *Psychoanalytic Studies of the Personality.* London: Routledge, p. 60.

19. Ibid., p. 31.

20. Ibid., p. 132.

21. Ibid., p. 65.
22. Winnicott, D.W. (1960). The theory of the parent–infant relationship. *International Journal of Psychoanalysis*, 41: 585–595.
23. Balint, M. (1979). *The Basic Fault*. London/New York, NY: Tavistock Publications.
24. Ibid., p. 22.
25. Ibid., p. 21.
26. Ibid., p. 132.
27. Ogden, T.H. (1983). The concept of internal object relations. *International Journal of Psychoanalysis*, 64: 227–241.
28. Ibid., p. 235.
29. Ogden, T.H. (1994). The analytic third: working with intersubjective clinical facts. *International Journal of Psychoanalysis*, 75: 3–19.
30. Young-Bruehl, E. (2011). Psychoanalysis and social democracy: a tale of two developments *Contemporary Psychoanalysis* 47: 179–203.
31. Ibid.
32. Kohut, H. (1971). *The Analysis of the Self*. Madison, CT: International Universities Press.
33. Winnicott, D.W. (1960). The theory of the parent–infant relationship. *International Journal of Psychoanalysis*, 41: 585–595.
34. Kohut, H. (1975). The future of psychoanalysis. *Annual Psychoanalysis*, 3: 325–340.
35. Kohut, H. (1972). Thoughts on narcissism and narcissistic rage. *Psychoanalytic Study of the Child*, 27: 360–400.
36. Lindon, J. (1994). Gratification and provision in psychoanalysis: should we get rid of "the rule of abstinence?" *Psychoanalytic Dialogues*, 4(4): 549–582.
37. Kohut, H. (1973). Psychoanalysis in a troubled world. *Annual Psychoanalysis*, 1: 3–25.
38. Murray, H.A. (1981). *Endeavors in Psychology: Selections from the Personology of Henry A. Murray*. New York, NY: Harper Collins.
39. Atwood, G.E., & Stolorow, R.D. (2014). *Structures of Subjectivity: Explorations in Psychoanalytic Phenomenology (Second Edition)*. New York, NY: Routledge.
40. Atwood, G.E., & Stolorow, R.D. (1992). *Contexts of Being: The Intersubjective Foundations of Psychological Life*. New York, NY: Routledge, p. 31.
41. Stolorow, R.D. (2015). A phenomenological-contextual, existential, and ethical perspective on emotional trauma. *Psychoanalytic Review*, 102(1): 123–138. Doi: dx.doi.org/10.1521/prev.2015.102.1.123.

42. Baranger, M., & Baranger, W. (2009). Spiral process and the dynamic field. In L.G. Fiorini (Eds.), *The Work of Confluence: Listening and Interpreting in the Psychoanalytic Field*. London: Karnac, pp. 45–61. (Original work published in 1979.)

43. Galatzer-Levy, R.M. (1995). Psychoanalysis and dynamical systems theory: prediction and self-similarity. *Journal of the American Psychoanalytic Association*, 43: 1085–1113.

44. Greenberg, J.R., & Mitchell, S.A. (1983). *Object Relations in Psychoanalytic Theory*. Cambridge, MA: Harvard University Press.

45. Ibid., p. 20.

46. Ibid., p. 20.

47. Klein, G.S.E. (1976). *Psychoanalytic Theory: An Exploration of Essentials*. New York, NY: International Universities Press.

48. Szasz, T. (1988). *The Ethics of Psychoanalysis: The Theory and Method of Autonomous Psychotherapy*. Syracuse, NY: University of Syracuse Press, p. 31.

49. Greenberg, J.R., & Mitchell, S.A. (1983). *Object Relations in Psychoanalytic Theory*. Cambridge, MA: Harvard University Press, p. 407.

50. Hoffman, I.Z. (1991). Discussion: toward a social-constructivist view of the psychoanalytic situation. *Psychoanalytic Dialogues*, 1(1): 74–105.

51. Renik, O. (1993). Analytic interaction: conceptualizing technique in light of the analyst's irreducible subjectivity. *Psychoanalytic Quarterly*, 62: 553–571.

52. Winnicott, D.W. (1965). The maturational processes and the facilitating environment. *International Psychoanalytic Library*, 64: 1–276. London: The Hogarth Press and the Institute of Psycho-Analysis, p. 186.

53. Baranger, M., & Baranger, W. (2009). Spiral process and the dynamic field. In L.G. Fiorini (Eds.), *The Work of Confluence: Listening and Interpreting in the psychoanalytic Field*. London: Karnac, pp. 45–61. (Original work published in 1979.)

CHAPTER 5

Creating the transformational frame

F reshly exposed to the philosophy underlying depth psychoanalytic work, and introduced to psychoanalysis' long and winding history, I explain another crucial contextual feature before
we embark on exploring the three metaphors guiding clinical work.
Framing psychoanalytic relationships is always delicate, sometimes
difficult, and occasionally dangerous. Jung referred to psychoanalysis as occurring within a crucible, and he used alchemical analogies
when describing the process. What transpires within the confines of
the psychoanalytic consulting room? How do the same four walls, the
same carpeted floor, and a similar configuration of furnishings create
sanctuary? Even after practicing for more than three decades, I still
feel surprise when individuals reveal their deepest personal feelings,
often entangled with deep feelings of shame, within the first few minutes of their first sessions. Depth psychotherapists provide patients
with a unique kind of environment—container, crucible, vessel,
space—inviting them to emotionally expose themselves.

The basics of framing depth psychotherapy relationships

Because psychoanalysts lack technology, formal procedures, or algorithmic methods that naturally create them, defining boundaries around psychoanalytic relationships can be difficult. Physicians don white coats with stethoscopes draped over their shoulders when encountering their patients who wait naked but for an examining gown. Attorneys greet clients while dressed in business attire, seated across desks in offices adorned with wall-to-wall books, legal journals, and stacks of case files. Psychoanalysts, in contrast, meet patients in more of a den-like setting, inviting them into an almost absurd, structured interpersonal relationship.

During psychoanalysis' early years, framing was easier. Psychoanalysts maintained boundaries much like how physicians did. They assumed the authority granted them by their social role. Patients enjoyed a fairly unequivocal sense of a diminished status, i.e., ill, needy, insane. Also, the almost universal use of the couch by early psychoanalysts signified their roles. Only patients lay on the couch. As psychoanalysis evolved, such easily definable social roles became blurred. Concepts like the corrective emotional experience, Kohut's "transmuting internalization," and Lindon's "optimal provision" complicated framing processes. These concepts require depth psychotherapists to account for where their caring for patients fits into the frame. They allowed for expressions of warmth, or more self-disclosures than traditionally thought acceptable. Some psychoanalysts influenced by these trends struggled to prevent their work from devolving into a variation of rent-a-friend.

Psychotherapeutic boundaries are the topic of endless papers and books in psychoanalysis, but they really need not be so complex. Virtually all practitioners believe they are establishing the "mutual but asymmetrical"[1] intimacy proposed by Aron—but with distinct limits. Psychoanalytic processes often become highly emotional, with patients becoming enraptured, enraged, or detached from the practitioners they consult. This is why prohibitions against touch prove so important. Interestingly, boundaries themselves often facilitate such emotions emerging, not to mention memories, thoughts, attitudes, and more. The frame contains these strong feelings, allowing them to be experienced and discussed, without being enacted physically. Unfortunately, sexual activity between psychotherapists and patients is not uncommon. Some estimates suggest it occurs in 10 percent of cases. I consider any overtly sexual enactment the same as sexual molestation: The patient is always in the more emotionally vulnerable position. Sexual behavior in psychoanalysis, then, is exploitative. It is extremely damaging to patients. The story of my work with Gilda, peppered through these pages, reveals how close I came to violating even physical boundaries.

Precisely because of the emotional vulnerability of patients, psychoanalysts ideally start sessions promptly, and they end them just as promptly. The starting point is easy to achieve; the ending not so much. Stolorow, already mentioned many times, once remarked that depth psychotherapists spend entire days telling their patients—who usually are closely attached to them—to "get out!" It is awkward, and even harmful, to abruptly end sessions during an emotionally intense moment. Competent framing allows for *some* flexibility in this regard. Each session is like a fractal, a slice of a patient's life. The regularity of session length creates a cadence over time. Along these lines, some practitioners of Lacanian analysis utilize scansion, or variable-length sessions, in working with patients. A scholar of Lacan, Bruce Fink, notes how, rather than stop psychoanalytic processes at an arbitrary ending point at 45 or 50 minutes, "we stop or 'scand' the session immediately after the significant formulation." The idea eliminates the tyranny of the clock, allowing patients to exit after receiving a meaningful interpretation or having an emotionally transformative experience. Fink adds, "instead of continuing while the patient says something highly significant, or allow them to bury a meaningful phrase under things of lesser importance, the psychoanalyst stops the session."[2] Such session endings emphasize work accomplished rather than duration. Lacan meant to punctuate each transformational experience. However, given the context of our capitalist society, and the fact that we psychoanalysts are selling a time-based service, this Lacanian technique is problematic. In my view, fairly firm time boundaries actually help with the transformational process; patients become accustomed to how long encounters last, and sink into them, knowing an end-point approaches. Once a course of sessions is underway, patients tend to adapt to the rhythm of the sessions.

Another theme in boundary maintenance concerns out-of-session contacts. These inevitably occur, particularly if depth psychotherapists live in the same area where they practice. Usually, clinicians wait and see if patients approach them in public in order to protect their privacy. Personally, I have no problem with a friendly encounter with a patient who approaches me, but I will strive to keep the meeting short. Why? To maintain the sanctity of the psychoanalytic process. We depth psychotherapists are not friends with our patients. Reality always threatens to impede psychotherapeutic processes, and friendship often beckons as one of the more common ways. Some patients unconsciously seek a friendship-like connection to avoid encountering any number of painful, difficult topics. Competent depth psychotherapy involves keeping a certain pressure up during and between sessions, a force that creates an intimate, bounded, and exploratory discourse.

Another element of framing concerns how sessions themselves are structured. The more conservative psychoanalysts will wait until patients speak to begin sessions. Their intention? To avoid guiding the patient. However, in actual practice, such an approach may come off as rudeness, and can even be traumatic. If patients greet me with a phrase like, "how are you?" which is common, I often reply "fine" or "OK," escort them into the consulting room, and stay quiet. I patiently wait and see what they do then. If a long silence ensues, I will usually initiate some contact by saying something like "where are you at?" or "how is your soul?" a phrase my patients learn represents an inquiry seeking information about what lurks beneath the surface of their thoughts.

Perhaps the most controversial boundary issue surrounds the question of self-disclosure. Conservative psychoanalysts say almost nothing about themselves. In one famous historical incident, a psychoanalyst who was a concentration camp survivor had a patient who suffered similarly. She expressed curiosity regarding the psychoanalysts' history in this regard. He refused to answer the question. The logic? Depth psychotherapists should remain focused on their patients' experiences. Their own experience is of no relevance. In the more modern approaches, specifically the intersubjective or relational approaches, the "real" relationship is considered an active part of the work. Depth psychotherapists, in a similar situation, would disclose their history of imprisonment. Risk exists on both sides of the self-disclosure debate:

Too little risks harming the patient, and too much blurs boundaries. In any event, self-disclosure should always be used sparingly, and always with the patient's best interest in mind.

Analogies between theater and psychoanalytic work

Although depth psychotherapy is often classified as an allied medical profession, practitioners typically veer way past symptom reduction. Depth psychotherapy processes are, in my view, a form of performance art.[3] They intend to transform patients, much like how theater affects audiences. Theater provides a number of useful metaphors for describing how depth psychotherapists manage the transformative elements of their work. When patrons attend theatrical performances, they select seats (spontaneously or purchased in advance). Their seats typically separate them from the stage by a gap or cordon of some type. Audience members know they are precluded from walking onto the stage. They know they will have no physical contact with the cast members. Like depth psychotherapy patients, they, too, have some expectation of how long the performance will last. These features mimic the framing of the psychoanalytic relationships. In many ways, depth psychotherapy unfolds like a play with only two participants to it.

Unlike actual theater, though, the roles played by the parties vary. Fairly consistently, clinicians serve as producers. They set the fee, sometimes in consultation with their patients. They certainly set the location. They remain in charge of the set design since they own or rent the "theaters" in which depth psychotherapy occurs. However, the role of director may be assumed by either party. Sometimes, when patients project their injured selves into the practitioners, they assume agency for the directorial role. They *direct* the course the process takes. Henrich Racker[4] invented the phrase, *concordant countertransference*, to describe what occurs when clinicians share the experience of their patients. Depth psychotherapists may feel small, weak, and inadequate, and they may perceive their patients as criticizing them—in a manner repeating patients' experiences with their parents. In these situations, clinicians identify with the self of the patients. Alternatively, they may experience what Racker termed *complementary countertransference*, meaning they assume the role, through projective identification, of the internal objects of patients. Practitioners themselves may begin to feel critical, judgmental, or otherwise negative toward patients. In such cases, they assume the role of archaic, internalized others in patients' minds. As depth psychotherapeutic processes unfold, clinicians ultimately play multiple roles—director, actor, and audience member. Even their primary role as producer can become fluid in that patients can fail to appear, show up late, or abruptly quit the shared performance.

Legal and ethical implications of framing

Various controversies regarding the degree of warmth, self-disclosure, and related framing themes are integrated within the realms of law and ethics. In the state of California, for example, the privacy and confidentiality of psychotherapy relationships are codified in the evidence code as well as in the range of regulations governing mental health professions. The evidence code arguably proves most relevant because it governs what law enforcement, prosecutors, and other government officials can access when seeking "evidence" related to a crime or lawsuit. California Evidence Code 1014, for example, establishes the "psychotherapist–patient privilege." The holder of the privilege is the person legally able to reveal information about a psychoanalysis. The law reads that

> the patient, whether or not a party [to the legal proceeding], has a privilege to disclose, and to prevent another from disclosing, a confidential communication between patient and psychotherapist if said privilege is claimed by a. the holder of the privilege; b. a person authorized to claim the privilege by the holder of the privilege, or c. the person who was the psychotherapist at the time of the confidential communication ...

In effect, patients control the power to withhold psychotherapeutic information from others. Even the US Supreme Court upholds the sanctity of depth psychotherapy relationships. In *US Supreme Court Jaffee v. Redmond* (95–266), 518 US 1 (1996), the privacy of the psychotherapeutic frame was validated:

Effective psychotherapy ... depends upon an atmosphere of confidence and trust in which the patient is willing to make a frank and complete disclosure of facts, emotions, memories, and fears. Because of the sensitive nature of the problems for which individuals consult psychotherapists, disclosure of confidential communications made during counseling sessions may cause embarrassment or disgrace. For this reason, the mere possibility of disclosure may impede development of the confidential relationship necessary for successful treatment.

Unusual in legal contracts, depth psychotherapists must adhere to a requirement that they maintain confidentiality, in perpetuity, *even* regarding the relationship itself. Psychoanalysts who may have not seen patients for years, or even decades, remain responsible for maintaining the privacy of whatever was discussed. Certain exceptions exist, but a complete description of them would require another book. Suffice to say that confidentiality must be broken in cases of child abuse, lethal threats made to others, or certain other extreme situations. These exceptions are rare, represent societal concerns overshadowing individual needs, and are controversial because of the damage which occurs whenever the frame must be invaded.

How framing works

Typically, depth therapists frame their professional relationships indirectly, simply through their behavior. Most orient patients new to the experience, showing them how to use the annunciator light, setting session times, and explaining, briefly, how psychoanalytic processes work. Part of facilitating transformational processes requires some mystery. An in-depth explanation, like I provide in these pages, might inhibit a patient—particularly a person who has never consulted a psychoanalyst before. Providing "informed consent" usually includes cost, fees for late cancelations, and billing information. Most often, this proves sufficient. In patients with more severe psychopathology, such as those with borderline personality disorders, defensive maneuvers may disrupt framing processes. These individuals are, by definition, unstable in mood and behavior. They are prone to fits of rage.

They might view their psychoanalysts as loving and friendly one week, and as angry and rejecting the next. Regarding framing specifically, they might push for physical contact, such as regular hugs or other forms of touch; they might make personal inquiries about their psychoanalysts' lives.

Naturally, boundary maintenance is of extreme importance in these cases—even though it might provoke these patients. Depth psychotherapists might need to directly instruct patients about the logic of bound aries and other framing behaviors. Interestingly, such problems with framing often end up providing grist for the psychoanalytic mill. Their mental pain and instability seep into other boundaries in their lives, manifesting, for example, in running late for work, becoming pathologically jealous in romantic relationships, or in poor self-care. Framing becomes part of the process of reining such primitive mental content back into the consulting room. These types of persons, in general, need help to digest their raw emotional material so that they can re-incorporate it into themselves in a less chaotic fashion. Maintaining the frame creates the container for these integrative processes to occur.

Michael Balint[5] differentiated between patients who display regression in the interest of recognition, called benign regression, and those regressing for instinctual gratification, known as malignant regression. The latter, occurring more commonly in patients with borderline or psychotic disorders, refers to the difficulty these patients have managing the psychoanalytic frame. As previously stated, Lacan[6] considers all desire as ultimately a desire for unconditional love. Patients may become distressed by the limits on psychoanalytic relationships, hoping to obtain unconditional love from their psychoanalysts. Because of the intimacy involved in psychoanalytic encounters, regardless of how asymmetrical they may be, patients sometimes become confused regarding boundaries. Again, boundaries create crucibles to explore any confusion emerging. And Balint's differentiation offers guidance for practitioners.

Some professional constraints are obvious. For example, most depth psychotherapists would agree that engaging in dual relationships with patients violates the psychoanalytic frame. Even novice psychoanalysts understand that having coffee with patients, employing them as their personal assistants, or otherwise involving them in social roles that parallel their patient role causes confusion that hampers, if not destroys, psychoanalytic processes. Many scholars, with Gabbard and Lester[7] among the most notable, write extensively about boundary mainte- nance. They helpfully distinguish between *boundary crossings*—defined as departures from the typical professional frame that are harmless, non-exploitative, and possibly even helpful—and *boundary violations* that harm patients. Ironically, I crossed boundaries myself, with Gilda, and provide you with reasons why and how I re-established the frame with her in later chapters.

Freud himself acknowledged how psychoanalytic work depends upon "the personal relation between the two people involved."[8] He emphasizes its humanism, its essential relational character, and by implication, the importance of binding the relationship. Psychoanalysts may utilize *framing* behaviors in the service of repairing previous inter- personal trauma. Even conservative psychoanalysts, devoted to absti- nence and neutrality, interrupt transference enactments and interpret them. Even those disagreeing with the more relational turn still behave a certain way, within the confines of the psychoanalytic relationship, to effect change. They bring transference, the repetition compulsion, and the meaning of dreams and other signs of the unconscious to patients' conscious awareness. They might eschew self-disclosure or expression of warmth toward patients, but they still utilize the psychodynamic relationship as the primary vehicle of change. They decline invitations by patients to behave in previously familiar, interpersonal ways.

More liberal practitioners tend to use their subjectivities as part of the mutative process. They may utilize various degrees of self- disclosure or directly express care or concern. Theorists such as Boesky[9] proposed that countertransference enactments, often including bound- ary crossings, may actually signal the *start* of a true psychoanalytic process. In other words, some boundary crossings are inevitable. How psychoanalysts manage these become part and parcel of their work. I demonstrate the unique, artistic quality of framing psychoanalytic relationships using specific examples from my work with Carlos, Gilda, and Penn.

Practitioners who prefer to work more formally, and who value abstinence and neutrality, typically structure their psychoanalytic rela- tionships and engage their patients differently than those preferring the more relational, interpersonal methods. They might decorate their offices sparsely. They tend to be more precise about session starting and ending times. Those more influenced by relational methods may create a greater sense of safety and comfort in the way they furnish their offices. Differences also exist outside of this one continuum. For example, psychoanalysts influenced by the Jungian tradition might display paintings, statues, or other objects intended to elicit mythic, archetypal themes from patients. In the final analysis, each psychoanalyst, facilitating his or her own unique version of the transformational process due to personality, style, cultural, and other factors, offers transformational encounters within clear boundaries, externally (as in an office setting and regular appointment times) and internally (as in the degree of warmth or self-disclosure). Framing professional relationships occurs regardless of psychoanalytic models of mind or practice. It requires the same kind of creativity inherent in all aspects of psychoanalytic work.

Pushing neutrality to excess

My training analyst—the depth psychotherapist I consulted four or five times a week while going through psychoanalytic training—showed remarkable conservatism when I saw him in the 1990s. He often sat silently during sessions. He offered few reactions, and he rarely displayed empathy for my emotional states. The memory reminds me of the joke that, in the first year of a Freudian analysis, an entire year could pass before the patient discovers her psychoanalyst died. (The other half of the joke is that it may take Kleinian psychoanalysts, known for making excessive interpretations, a year to realize their *patient* has died.) I quickly learned how, despite his interpersonal coldness, he at least listened carefully. He remembered nearly everything I said. In this manner, he showed a degree of devotion to me, even caring. However, the emotionality ended there. On one occasion, well before Al Gore invented the internet, I asked him if I could borrow an issue of *The New Yorker* from his waiting room. I prefaced the request with an acknowledgment that, if he kept past issues in a binder, took them home to his wife, or otherwise held onto them, I would withdraw my request. He failed to respond to my question. Instead, he interpreted my behavior, asking:

"Do you think your request could reflect a sense of entitlement?"

"No," I replied.

Had I *expected* to be given the issue, stolen it, or not asked him in a considerate manner, then perhaps I had been entitled. But I did none of those things. At the end of that month, when I handed him the monthly payment for services he rendered, I wrote a check for $5 short of the total. A few days earlier, I went to the bank in my building where I had the $5 converted into a roll of nickels. I handed him the check with the coin roll, and quipped,

"This is so you never forget the impact of depriving me of *The New Yorker* issue."

The psychoanalyst said nothing in response to that behavior, even though I was overtly hostile. Practicing in the more liberal, relational manner myself, I would happily give leftover magazines to patients. However, I might still interpret the request if relevant, e.g., "can I take all the magazines in your waiting room?" Similarly, I would explore the behavior of a patient who reported wishing for a magazine issue but feeling afraid of asking for it. Some conservative psychoanalysts still deny the gratification of any patient's wishes, however small. I respectfully disagree. I had never asked my training analyst for anything before, paid his fee regularly, and dutifully attended the training analysis for years. As Ferenczi argued in his paper "Confusion of tongues,"[10] the incident symbolizes deeper themes and, in my case certainly, the use of neutrality was injurious.

Pushing relationality to excess

Greenberg coined the phrase "psychoanalytic excess,"[11] extending Freud's original phrase, "therapeutic ambition,"[12] to refer to taking the caring environment of relationally oriented psychoanalysts too far. Some poorly trained depth psychotherapists confuse facilitating transformational encounters with friendship. The difference is crucial. While depth psychotherapists ideally create a welcoming, friendly environment, they cannot act as friends with their patients. Another relational psychoanalyst, Aron, encourages his patients to disclose to him anything they observe about *him*, writing,

I often ask patients to speculate or fantasize about what is going on inside of me, and in particular I focus on what patients have noticed about my internal conflicts ... I assume that the patient may very well have noticed my anger, jealousy, excitement, or whatever before I recognize it in myself.[13]

Aron's reputation remains excellent, but I wonder about the extremity of the invitation. Why assume patients understand my conflicts before I do? Why nudge them to focus on me? Certainly, my subjectivity plays a role in my psychoanalytic relationships, but the work must remain asymmetrical.

In his passionate critique of the relational approaches, Jon Mills—a self-proclaimed relational analyst himself, and now a dear friend—also warns of the risk of its excesses. He describes how these approaches allow for:

malleability in the treatment frame, selectivity in interventions that are tailored to the unique needs and qualities of each patient, and a proper burial of the prototypic solemn analyst who is fundamentally removed from relating as one human being to another in the service of a withholding, frustrating, and ungratifying methodology designed to provoke transference enactments, deprivation, and unnecessary feelings of rejection, shame, guilt, and rage.[14]

As noted repeatedly, like a sinner seeking redemption, I soon share the ways work with Gilda bent the frame to a near-breaking point. Mills continues, following in the footsteps of Hegel and Whitehead,[15] to describe how depth psychotherapy facilitates patients' *process of becoming*. The relational approaches encourage mutuality—a concept frequently misunderstood. Mutuality does not mean equality, or the loss of proper framing processes. It encourages psychoanalysts to become more vulnerable and engaged while still retaining the asymmetry, or what Mills calls "proportional exchange." He adds,

within the consulting room there is generally more dialogue rather than monologue, less interpretation and more active attunement to the process within the dyad, more emphasis on

affective experience over conceptual insight, and more interpersonal warmth conveyed by the analyst, thus creating a more
emotionally satisfying climate for both involved.[16]

Thomas Szasz once quipped that depth psychotherapists should greet
each patient with one and only one need in mind: *Their need for money.*

The position is a bit extreme, perhaps even crass. Nonetheless, he
makes an important point. Psychoanalysts sell a service, and they
expect payment for it. If they are primarily channeling their need to
rescue, to love, to parent, or to salve, or to literally serve as a surrogate
lover to their patients, they fail them. No matter how relational or interpersonal the model of psychotherapeutic change, the doctor remains
the doctor and the patient remains the patient.

Many fear that Jody Davies, for example, showed therapeutic excess
when describing a case involving a "mutually constructed, intersubjective engaged playground" featuring "interaction between two actively
engaged participants."[17] Her controversial 1994 paper, titled "Love in
the afternoon," included descriptions of her sharing her sexual fantasies about a male patient. She considered the self-disclosures imperative in helping him view himself as attractive. Did she stray too far?
The question remains open. Because the psychoanalytic frame deliberately invites patients into the more regressed position, someone must
captain the ship. Piloting becomes crucial when sailing into broiling,
unstable waters involving sexuality. Mills considers Davies' approach
an example of therapeutic excess. I have little basis for criticizing Davies
myself because, at times anyway, I lost sight of the process. I too failed
in proper navigation. The following clinical examples demonstrate how
the more relational, interpersonal approaches can be used, and sometimes abused, even by experienced clinicians like myself.

Problems in framing psychoanalysis with Carlos

My work with Carlos provides multiple examples of how framing processes became a central part of our work together. As I described previously, he walked into my consulting room boldly idealizing me while
also requesting a multiple-session-per-week psychoanalytic process.
I did not have four appointment times open, and so I started him on
once-weekly sessions and offered him cancelations to ensure we had at

least two sessions per week. He arrived punctually, if not early, for these meetings. He remained eager for a "formal psychoanalysis." Within two months, I had made four sessions each week, on four different days, available. After another few months, Carlos' resistance to emotional exposure first presented itself. Carlos requested he be provided with two double sessions, complaining that the four 45-minute-long meetings were too short for him to "get deep." After much discussion, including how the arrangement deviated from how a formal psychoanalysis is viewed, I relented. I arranged for him to have the two double appointments he requested. After another few months, Carlos began to indirectly retreat. He canceled some appointments. He arrived late for others. Sometimes, he showed up as much as thirty or even 45 minutes late, relegating his double appointments to single ones.

I remember reacting with guilt, irritation, and even anger at his avoidance behaviors. I interpreted their meaning, and Carlos readily agreed he feared "too much pain." Meanwhile, he eagerly paid for the appointments, even if he missed them altogether (which was part of our contractual agreement). Why the guilt? Because Carlos, highly financially successful despite little formal education, paid my fee while I made phone calls, sent emails, and even worked on this book. The irritation I felt was in reaction to his interference with the psychoanalytic process. He had, in effect, placed me on a "retainer" in which he could maintain the illusion of undergoing psychoanalysis while, in fact, remaining relatively invulnerable. Consistent with his defensive style, he often also ended sessions early—all in accordance with how he wanted to run things. He might say, with 10 or 15 minutes remaining in the session, something like, "It's not that I don't love you, Alan, but I need to go recruit more salespeople." He would then stand up, warmly shake my hand, collect his keys and the mobile phone he left on the table near the door, and rush out. As the patterns solidified, I felt increasingly frustrated and out of control. More relevant to the *Exorcist* chapter, his behavior illustrates projective identification. Carlos unconsciously triggered in me the vulnerable feelings that he was, to use the Kleinian phrase, evacuating into me.

Carlos interfered with framing limits in other ways. Early on, he predicted that, someday, I would "throw out" my professional ethics and meet him for a drink. Meanwhile, he reacted to my sudden medical leave in a manner unique in my practice. Of the many patients I abandoned when given literally 20 minutes to exit my practice, Carlos was the only one who, at least initially, refused to resume our sessions. When he ultimately returned, he assumed all theatrical roles: producer, director, actor, and audience. He insisted on speaking on the phone first, reduced the session frequency to one time per week, and asked for assurances he would be informed of any other future absences by me. For the duration of our second season—which began after my medical leave—Carlos was less trusting. He often arrived late. Although I had regained my health, Carlos feared abandonment again. He defended himself through hypervigilance, readying himself to leave me before I could leave him. In fact, after another year of weekly depth psychotherapy, he terminated the treatment. Carlos said he could not handle more exposure to his personal vulnerability. Perhaps he would have taken a break, and ended our "second season," anyway. However, and in retrospect, I suspect he experienced my medical crisis as traumatic. He was not able to recover. By reducing the session frequency for the next year, and then directing the therapy by ending it when he did, Carlos avoided vulnerability. His way of managing the frame of the psychotherapy exemplifies, rather dramatically, how framing processes become part and parcel of depth psychotherapy processes. Carlos later returned for a third season, by which point, it appeared, he felt more prepared to face the depth of his childhood trauma.

The perilous framing process with Gilda

My work with Gilda represents how the personal feelings of depth psychotherapists, their life situations, and the countertransference dynamically interact when framing psychoanalytic relationships. Gilda began consulting me literally two months after the worst medical misadventure of my life. Furthermore, my marriage had entered a rocky period itself—likely resulting from the incredible stress of the illness and the subsequent surgery. These factors likely contributed to my instantaneous attraction to her.

Depth psychotherapists are "fellow sufferers."[18] They travel through the twists and turns of their own lives, just like their patients do. They are anything but free of their own personality foibles. As described previously, I have a particular vulnerability to wishing to rescue others. The Jungians would describe such a tendency as a manifestation of the Great Mother archetype. Gilda had suffered depression since childhood, had been emotionally and sexually abused, struggled through a prolonged child custody battle with her recently estranged husband, and only barely coped with her new job as a research assistant. She needed help. Moreover, Gilda's former psychoanalyst, who referred her to me because of a terminal illness, died within the first year of my working with her.

In retrospect, the combination of my personal vulnerabilities, my feelings for Gilda, and the countertransference resulted in me crossing boundaries in terms of framing my professional relationship with her. Unlike the situation with Carlos in which framing irregularities were primarily caused by him, I was the primary one responsible for the problems in the professional relationship with Gilda. However, there were times she seemed to invite rescue. Also, she occasionally behaved seductively. For the most part, however, I was the one who strayed, distracted by the intensity of my feelings of powerlessness, my caring for Gilda, and my desire to rescue her.

The usual framing processes unfolded without difficulty until Gilda was assaulted around two years into our work together. The intensity of her distress, the lack of support from friends and family, and the severity of her symptoms—especially the psychogenic fugue states—contributed to my losing my footing. Rather than hospitalize her in a psychiatric facility, I encouraged Gilda to meet me six days a week. I had not previously offered such intensive treatment to any patient. Some colleagues might argue that seeing patients on weekends is seductive. It is traditional family time. It is time for romantic play with lovers or friends. However, and in my defense, I wished to prevent inpatient hospitalization. My gamble ultimately paid off, but only at the price of harming our professional relationship.

Other subtle alterations in the frame developed. I extended the length of sessions. I professed my strong personal feelings for her, specifically telling her how much I feared for her safety when she was out all hours of the night. I confessed how powerless I felt. Sometimes these frame-breaking behaviors, and excessive self-disclosures, were triggered by Gilda's distress. Other times, they occurred because of my own feelings of impotence. As I describe in more detail in the next chapter,

I ruptured the frame in other, more subtle ways, like by contacting other involved parties.

These boundary crossings all demonstrate how I became unequivocally overinvolved with Gilda. I thought I was the only person who understood her mental fragility. What had been a challenging psychotherapeutic situation due to her childhood trauma and my strong erotic countertransference rapidly transcended into one dominated by my own experience of her pain, my feelings of powerlessness, and my wish to rescue her. Several significant changes in Gilda's life made matters worse. Her daughter moved out, and Gilda felt abandoned. Also, because the psychogenic fugue states had lessened, and I felt increasingly uncomfortable with the six-day-per-week sessions, I reduced our meetings to five a week. Of course, she and I prepared for the session frequency reduction. We discussed the change for weeks in advance of its occurring. Despite the attention paid, Gilda regressed as soon as we started meeting less frequently. She re-experienced the acute symptoms of the PTSD, including the fugue states. To compensate for the reduced contact, I extended the length of the sessions from 45 to 60 minutes without increasing her fee. During this transition period, it felt like Gilda and I were wrestling to contain her regression.

The most extreme boundary crossing, and arguably a violation, occurred immediately after we started meeting less frequently. I employed Gilda to prepare some research proposals for me. The disability income she received amounted to less than half of her usual salary. Her financial situation deteriorated. To reduce her expenses, we reduced session frequency to three times a week. I lowered her fee again. Trying to help her financial situation, I paid Gilda for preparing four research proposals. Ironically, and an example of why so-called dual relationships prove so problematic, Gilda struggled to compose the proposals because of her ongoing distress. Within two months of this clearly unprofessional arrangement, I began to feel irritated. She prepared the grant proposals in a disorganized fashion. When I gently brought the mistakes to Gilda's attention, she reacted with anger. Notice how my roles as psychoanalyst and employer overlapped. When not annoyed, I felt guilty and ashamed. I knew the dual relationship was wrong, and that I had overstepped in trying to help her. Gilda and I discussed the situation in detail. When I told her I needed to end the employment arrangement, she became enraged. Gilda perceived the termination, after she had completed only two of the four proposals, as evidence I considered her incompetent. She felt betrayed.

The situation took one final dark turn before we, together, transitioned the professional relationship back into a proper frame. Gilda's daughter withdrew from her completely. Apparently, she, too, felt frightened by her distress and her powerlessness to help her mother. Gilda became even more withdrawn. Her already socially isolated, restricted lifestyle became more so. Ultimately, she became physically ill, developing a difficult-to-diagnose seizure disorder. She became suicidal. Gilda also began withdrawing from me. She canceled one or two of our three scheduled sessions per week; she asked to hold others by telephone. I considered insisting that she appear in person because I was concerned about the risk of suicide. At a point demarcating the bottom of this awful, almost-uncontrollable wave, I offered to pay Gilda a $400 advance payment for the two proposals she had yet to complete. I told her she need not complete them. The money was to pay for anti-seizure medication she could not afford. Feeling dizzy and ill, Gilda attended an in-person session to accept the payment. Clearly conflicted, she reluctantly accepted the cash-filled envelope.

Handing Gilda the money—reminiscent of an illicit drug deal—struck me like a bolt of lightning. In that precise moment, I fully realized the degree to which I lost control of our relationship. I contacted a senior colleague who agreed to consult with me about the situation. I began meeting with her, once weekly, and we continued to meet for the next six months. She validated my excessive involvement, helped me understand the various factors (personal, countertransference-related, and Gilda's part), and guided me back into the proper professional role. She offered helpful advice regarding how my need to rescue had meshed so well with Gilda's truly dire situation.

As I began to restore the psychoanalytic relationship, Gilda remained enraged with me. She was furious I terminated the employer-employee relationship. Whereas she previously had difficulty accessing the anger she felt at how she was abused as a child, at the other men who exploited her, at her assailants, and at the research institute which abandoned her, her hostility toward me emerged with fiery intensity. Many sessions consisted of her simply shouting at me, delineating the many ways I failed her. She raged at me for "giving in" to her seductiveness.

She accused me of lacking empathy for her situation: impoverished, alone, and disabled.

Despite her withering accusations, I remained steadfast in repairing the frame. In fact, I held to it with renewed vigor—despite Gilda's intense reactions. I refrained from overtly reacting. I responded with empathy to her intense emotional states but without any additional self-disclosures. I helped her to clarify her feelings. As she became calmer, I interpreted the rescue–victim dynamic, explaining the deeper, sado-masochistic contractual level and its tendency to reverse. In fact, the reversal was most evident during this period of her anger at me: I became the weak, incompetent, injured party and Gilda the triumphant abuser-of-me. I initially fell into the narcissistic role by entertaining omnipotent beliefs I could rescue her and, when Gilda later transitioned into intense angry feelings at me, our roles reversed. I took full responsibility for my behaviors. I admitted my error in employing her and giving her the $400. I fully and unconditionally apologized for what was "purely my error."

Over the ensuing months, Gilda's anger gradually subsided. We discussed, more carefully this time, what fee would work given her current financial situation. We agreed upon a new fee, and we also reduced the session frequency to twice a week. I kept to our newly agreed-upon fee. Perhaps because Gilda and I had already spent so much time discussing her reaction to the session frequency, she adjusted well to the reduced frequency. I continued to spend a full hour meeting with her during these twice-weekly depth psychotherapy sessions.

The transition period lasted around six months. In retrospect, I believe my post-surgical vulnerability, as well as the marital disharmony associated with it, contributed to my loss of judgment. The abruptness of the assault on Gilda had mixed, in an explosive way, with my personal life concerns. I kept these realizations to myself, simply telling Gilda on several occasions, "I understand I let my own vulnerabilities interfere with our work."

Away from sessions, I worked through my own feelings, including some anger I felt toward Gilda. I look back on the months of fee reductions, and on my having employed Gilda, with embarrassment. I also feel some anger at allowing myself to, in a certain way, be exploited. Rather than act out against her, I channeled my irritation into restoring the psychoanalytic frame. Gilda continued to meet with me twice-weekly for three more years. She ultimately recovered from the shock of the assault. She obtained an editing position at a different firm. Our relationship terminated in a positive way. We spent several months reviewing the "long and strange trip" we journeyed on together, summarized what she had learned about herself and her relationships, and set an end date well in advance. Ultimately, the psychoanalytic process ended in a positive way. However, those last few years felt like an extremely rough ride for both of us.

The straightforward framing processes with Penn

I fear I deny Penn sufficient attention because, unlike Carlos or Gilda, my work with him offers few illustrations of problems with framing. And how could he possibly compete with the near-disastrous framing difficulties I encountered with Gilda? Penn displayed one subtle problem, though, and it haunted our professional relationship for the first few years. We established a positive rapport quickly. Penn, a young man when we first met, had no experience with any kind of psychotherapy. Soon, he became acquainted with the dance of the work. We had two regular appointment times per week. His attendance was steady. A few months in, Penn began arriving late. His lateness became quickly predictable. He was rarely on time, but he was also rarely more than 10 minutes late. He arrived in a rush, apologized for his tardiness, and then described whatever was on his mind at the time. Typical of psychoanalysts of any theoretical orientation, I made inquiries regarding possible meanings of the tardiness. Penn and I both considered various hypotheses. Ultimately, we agreed that, to use his words, he "distrusted the reception." He could not *believe* I would find him interesting, be curious about his life, or empathize with his emotions.

Over the course of the ensuing months, we developed a shared understanding of the process, which, in many ways, mimicked the way he ran his life. Penn had never fully recovered from the injuries sustained from his "always angry, raging" mother. He turned inward, and assumed a pseudo-mature stance. He considered himself personally responsible for whatever love and comfort he might receive. Much of his academic, occupational, and financial success followed from such excessive self-sufficiency. Predictably, Penn had consistently struggled in the realm of interpersonal intimacy. The stereotypical "alpha male," brightly emerging once he completed his professional training, was displayed in his lecturing, teaching, mentoring, and writing. He easily *gave* love and attention to others; he struggled to *receive* it. It only followed a performance, or so he believed. Over the years, he became "worn out" by the constant pressure to perform. Many years of interpretations of the phenomenon and of confrontations of how it served to protect him from his vulnerability followed. Gradually, his lateness lessened from 5 to 4 to 3 to 2 to 1 minute. Eventually, he began arriving at sessions in a timely manner and, as I describe in the next chapter, actually started arriving early so he could sink into the discomfort of *being* as opposed to *doing*.

Hopefully, it has now become clear how framing processes proved a foundational part of my work with Carlos, Gilda, and Penn. For Carlos, it revealed the threat of interpersonal vulnerability and how he continually strived to reverse it. For Gilda, the framing process revealed my own vulnerability (ironically) rather than hers. As I noted, Gilda's own personal style, and her mental pain, also invited me to deviate from proper professional boundaries. Ideally, I could have simply observed them, interpreted them, and not enacted them. But I did, and the memory still haunts me. My errors ended up opening a possibility for more growth, but such positive change could have occurred without my problematic enactments. For Penn, the framing process served as a projection screen for his own discomfort at receiving love and attention. It offered both of us a way to enhance his self-understanding and his tolerance for mental pain. Eventually, the combination of insight, combined with his exposure to the emotional discomfort around which his entire character was structured, allowed him to face, and ultimately reduce, the pain of early childhood trauma.

Finding the balance

Much of depth psychoanalytic work requires artistry. Finding the balance between excessive neutrality and excessive warmth proves difficult. Even Freud equivocated on the point. Many depth psychotherapists believe Freud recommended psychoanalysts behave like blank screens to their patients, that the analyst should be opaque. In truth, he invoked the metaphor of the mirror—hardly the same meaning as blank or opaque. He intended depth psychotherapists to facilitate patients having a stark, honest view of themselves. And, yet, Freud fed some patients, lent money to others, and took still others on vacation with him.[19] He showed great kindness to many patients, calling into question just how well he shined the mirror of his own personality. No depth psychotherapist can provide the perfect mirror. Their values, biases, theoretical orientations, personal preferences, and more always break through whatever attempt they make at neutrality. Offering pure reflection to patients remains an aspirational goal, always guiding the work, but never fully achievable. As I have shown in describing framing processes, and using these three professional relationship as examples, framing indeed is a fundamental vehicle for introducing parts of patients' unconscious minds to them.

Mills again aptly describes the artistic balance between excessive neutrality and excessive intimacy, writing:

> Traditional approaches, whether intended or not, implicitly foster (if not encourage) a detached, scientific, experience-far observer paradigm, whereas the relational approach sees the inherent value of being real and genuine and fostering an experience-near, coparticipant observer stance, whereby the patient is related to as a nonobjectified person.[20]

On that clarifying note, I bring this discussion of boundaries to an end. I anticipated readers would require a sense of framing processes before I described more details of the actual clinical work, and I hope these last few chapters helped in this regard. Knowledge enhanced by understanding the philosophical and psychoanalytic background of the field, I added one more important preamble: the idea of framing. As the next chapter will reveal, framing plays the most crucial role when psychoanalysts assume the role of *Lover*. And it is to that metaphor that we now turn.

Notes

1. Aron, L. (1996). *A Meeting of Minds: Mutuality in Psychoanalysis*. New York, NY: The Analytic Press.
2. Fink, B. (2014). *Against Understanding: Cases and Commentary in a Lacanian Key* (Vol. 2). New York, NY: Routledge.
3. Karbelnig, A. (2014). The analyst is present: viewing the psychoanalytic process as performance art. *Psychoanalytic Psychology*, 33 (Supplement 1): 153–172. Doi: 10.1037/a0037332.
4. Racker, H. (1982). *Transference and Countertransference*. London: Routledge.
5. Balint (1979). *The Basic Fault: Therapeutic Aspects of Regression*. New York, NY: Brunner/Mazel.
6. Lacan, J. (2008). *My Teaching*. D. Macey (Trans.). New York, NY: Verso.
7. Gabbard, G.O., & Lester, E.P. (1995). *Boundaries and Boundary Violations in Psychoanalysis*. New York, NY: Basic Books.
8. Freud, S. (1916–1917). *Introductory Lectures On Psycho-Analysis. The Standard Edition of the Complete Psychological Works of Sigmund Freud, Volumes XV–XVI*. London: Hogarth Press, p. 441.
9. Boesky, D. (1990). The psychoanalytic process and its components. *Psychoanalytic Quarterly*, 59: 580–584.
10. Ferenczi, S. (1949). Confusion of the tongues between the adults and the child (the language of tenderness and of passion). *International Journal of Psychoanalysis*, 30: 225–230.
11. Greenberg, J. (2001). The analyst's participation. *Journal of the American Psychoanalytic Association*, 49(2): 359–381.
12. Freud, S. (1912e). Recommendations to physicians practicing psycho-analysis. *The Standard Edition of the Complete Psychological Works of Sigmund Freud, Volume XII (1911–1913): The Case of Schreber, Papers on Technique and Other Works*. London: Hogarth Press, pp. 109–120.
13. Aron, L. (1991). The patient's experience of the analyst's subjectivity. *Psychoanalytic Dialogues*, 1(1): 29–51.
14. Mills, J. (2012). *Conundrums: A Critique of Contemporary Psychoanalysis*. New York, NY: Routledge.
15. Whitehead, A.N. (1978). *Process and Reality*. (Corrected edition). New York, NY: Free Press.
16. Ibid., p. 97.

17. Davies, J. (1994). Love in the afternoon: a relational reconsideration of desire and dread. *Psychoanalytic Dialogues*, 4: 153–170.

18. Orange, D.M. (2011). *The Suffering Stranger: Hermeneutics for Everyday Clinical Practice and Everyday Life*. New York, NY: Routledge.

19. Freud, S. (1912). Recommendations to physicians practicing psycho-analysis. *The Standard Edition of the Complete Psychological Works of Sigmund Freud, Volume XII (1911–1913): The Case of Schreber, Papers on Technique and Other Works*. London: Hogarth Press, pp. 109–120.

20. Mills, J. (2011). *Conundrums: A Critique of Relational Psychoanalysis*. New York, NY, Routledge, p. 102.

CHAPTER 6

The *Lover*

Illusory or not, persons in love feel a blissful sense of mutual acceptance. The involved parties, enraptured, give unconditional care and acknowledgment to one another. The love for their beloved is pure, and the love of the other warms them like sunshine. While not as intense, psychoanalysts bring their *presence* to their patients in a way echoing how lovers treat one another. They offer deep levels of attention, curiosity, interest, and respect. They listen intensely. The psychoanalytic relationship itself influences patients' internal dramas, enhancing their sense of value and worth. More than just interpreting intense self-criticism, for example, depth psychotherapy structurally reshapes self-images. In this chapter, I explore how love is foundational to depth psychotherapy, including how psychodynamic clinicians manage the nuances of delivering such reparative caring.

Unlike the traditional attitude of the physician guided by scientism, psychoanalysts receive their patients' experiences as fully as possible. They metaphorically greet their patients with wide open arms. Whereas physicians may listen with a specific focus, i.e., delineating primary symptoms, their development, and contextual factors like immune vulnerabilities, psychoanalysts follow their patients' trains of thought and emotion. As time passes, and they hear the intimate details of patients' experiences, they begin caring. Such affection may not develop immediately. At various times, practitioners may hate their patients, fear them, or experience a range of negative emotions toward them. However, they cannot help but become emotionally involved with them.

In describing an ideal attitude for anthropologists studying foreign cultures, Clifford Geertz writes:

> Understanding the form and pressure of, to use the dangerous word one more time, natives' inner lives, is more like grasping a proverb, catching an allusion, seeing a joke—or, as I have suggested, reading a poem—that it is like achieving communion.[1]

Depth psychotherapists, too, seek communion with their patients. Their patients share incredibly intimate elements of their lives, from their fury at their uncles who abused them to their erotic lives with their boyfriends and more. The way clinicians' metaphorically unfold their wings to receive patients' experiences, week after week, month after month, creates safety, invites introspection, dissolves shame, and rebuilds, at least partially, the destruction of self-images caused by neglect, abuse, and other forms of trauma.

Freud and love

Freud considered feelings of love problematic by either party to the psychoanalytic encounter. He identified it as a form of resistance. To prevent it from contaminating the professional relationship, he emphasized "abstinence."[2] Depth psychotherapists, Freud believes, eschew receiving gratification from patients or delivering it to them. Patients pay psychotherapists for insight, and to strengthen the power of reason over the passions. Practitioners must remain as detached, scientific, and objective as possible. Any manifestation of love in the professional relationship, Freud believed, risks creating "wild analysis."[3] I remember a supervisee whose prior supervisor criticized her caring feelings, proclaiming: "Your job is to understand, not care." The prior supervisor had likely been swayed by the historical and sociocultural context of psychoanalysis' origins. I strongly disagreed, suggesting that patients' self-understanding is actually enhanced by caring.

In his "Observations on transference-love," Freud acknowledged, paradoxically, how frequently love enters depth psychotherapeutic relationships. He proposed the phrase, transference-love, as a way of identifying the phenomenon. He thought transference was a phenomenon resulting from patients projecting infantile desires onto their psychoanalysts. In essence, patients' internal dramas become entangled with their psychoanalytic relationships. Love is almost always a component of the transference. Rather than a simple appreciation for the service provided, patients might fall in love with their clinicians. Or they may imagine the love they never received from their parents, their siblings, their husbands, or wives emanates from their depth psychotherapists. Such yearning presents more intensely if patients' childhood featured deprivation.

On the one hand, Freud considered such manifestations of love as highly dangerous. He feared it impaired patients' incentive "to do work and to make changes," adding:

> And what we could offer would never be anything else than a surrogate, for the patient's condition is such that, until her repressions are removed, she is incapable of getting real satisfaction.[4]

In essence, Freud warns, patients may view them as lovers or parents, but these projections must be sloughed off. Years before the relational turn, Freud had not even imagined patients internalizing their psychoanalysts' caring for them. *Au contraire*, the psychoanalytic field required sterilization. Love in psychoanalysis was a kind of poison akin to bacteria contaminating a surgical field. Freud recommended depth psychotherapists prepare themselves for a "threefold battle"—against forces pulling the two parties toward a real interpersonal relationship, against opponents who deny the centrality of sexual instincts, and:

> against patients who at first behave like opponents but later on reveal the overvaluation of sexual life which dominates them, and who try to make [them] captive to their socially untamed passion.[5]

Here, Freud reveals his devotion to the power of *Eros* as a basic motivating force (his first proposed drive, followed later by the dual-drive model). By exposing their sexual urges, Freud feared, patients ensnare psychoanalysts. These worries, emerging at the height of the Victorian era in Europe, led Freud additionally to fear these phenomena would draw negative attention to the profession. He imagined the public would "doubtless seize upon this discussion of transference-love as another opportunity for directing the attention of the world to the serious danger of this therapeutic method."[6] Therefore Freud, unlike his mid-twentieth-century disciples, considered love dangerous and requiring vigilant management.

On the other hand, Freud paradoxically acknowledged the positive effects of love in transformative processes. He compares psychoanalysts to chemists working with highly explosive substances, asking:

> But when have chemists ever been forbidden, because of the danger, from handling explosive substances, which are indispensable, on account of their effects? … In medical practice there will always be room for the "*ferrum*" and the "*ignis*" side by side with the "*medicina*" and in the same way we shall never be able to do without a strictly regular, undiluted psychoanalysis which is not afraid to handle the most dangerous mental impulses and to obtain mastery over them for the benefit of the patient.[7]

In this excerpt, Freud correctly asserts that iron (methodology) and fire (love) closely co-exist. Contemporary psychoanalysts rarely concern themselves with "mastery of impulses" (although containing impulsive behavior could certainly become relevant depending on the individual psychoanalyst–patient relationship). Freud's anxiety over potential explosions in the realm of love was well-placed. It remains, in many ways, an ever-present risk. However, these manifestations are easily managed. Ironically, and as noted in the last chapter, Freud's case studies reveal his own deep care for his patients.

Influenced by Freud's love-anxiety, the other early pioneers of psychoanalysis also treated love in psychoanalytic relationships as potentially destabilizing. He and his early followers—mostly men, mostly physicians—feared love sounded unscientific. They worried it would harm their abilities to compete with their medical colleagues.

Most of all, they dreaded eliciting comparisons to faith healing or, worse, to prostitution—admittedly an awkward association but one which is, nonetheless, not without some merit. Ironically, and with more than a century passing since Freud's invention of the psychoanalytic profession, caring, listening, accepting, acknowledging, receiving, witnessing[8]—variations of loving—constitute the bedrock of depth psychotherapists' work. The now well-worn phrase, mutual but asymmetrical intimacy, refers, in part, to depth psychotherapists' presence: Intimacy means love; the asymmetry refers to framing processes described previously. Contemporary scholars studying early social interactions between infants and their caregivers use phrases like attachment theory[9] to provide scientific cover for what are, in essence, studies of loving relations. Their models validate how early familial relations create internal dramas; they also prove how psychoanalytic work alters them. However, attachment research only indirectly references the word "love." Scholars of attachment processes also fear love sounds too unscientific.

Freud's earliest treatment recommendations offer machine-like, technical, and even surgical metaphors. Words like ego, tortuously affected by internal forces emanating from the superego and the id, describe the self; words like object, self-object, internal object, and the like describe the way we carry images of others in our minds. These objects are altered by interactions with others and, more generally, culture. These configurations of self and other create the internal drama. However, and consistent with the zeitgeist of its formative era, the concept of an internal drama did not, and in many circles still does not, sound scientific enough. Therefore, ego became popularized, as did variations on the term object like rejecting, exciting, libidinal, and antilibidinal objects. These technical-sounding words and phrases intend to make the mind comport with scientism. Psychoanalysis remains mostly ensconced within this unfortunate prison, which blocks words like love, or even internal dramas, from entry.

Love, interpersonal contracts, and Greek philosophy

Anticipating the flood of objections to the heretical idea that love represents the foundation of psychoanalytic transformation, I suggest all relationships exist within overt or covert contracts. Married couples, for example, differ in the extent to which they tolerate the involvement of third parties. Some married persons are comfortable with their spouses working 60 hours per week, or spending two nights out a week with their friends; others prefer their marriage to dominate all other activities. Some couples socialize actively with others; others prefer spending most of their time with one another. In like manner, parents differ in their degrees of intimacy with their children. Some prefer more formal boundaries, even with their adult children. They avoid discussion of topics such as money or sex; others consider their children close friends. Friendships have the same range of intimacy, with some organized around a third entity, such as work, sports, or some other recreational activity, and others privileging the direct sharing of intimate thoughts and emotions.

Love inhabits almost every imaginable relationship, including feelings that employers have for employees or vice versa. Most educators feel love toward their students. Because of their imbalanced nature, the risk of exploitation lingers. Yet that risk does not eliminate the foundation of love on which these relationships rest. And, as noted, these professionals, like psychoanalysts, learn how to set boundaries and otherwise cope with love's emergence. The type of psychoanalytic presence previously described, while highly focused and intense, obviously comes with constraints. Framing requires depth psychotherapists to maintain unique, bounded, and professional relationships. Even if their patients fall into a state of despair—weeping, for example, or displaying intense emotional pain in any number of ways—depth psychotherapists will not sit on couches next to their patients, holding or touching them. Psychoanalytic love is subtle.

More primitively organized patients, or those who urgently seek love from their psychotherapists, bring unique challenges to the work. They may resent the abrupt manner in which sessions end; they may want more contact with their clinicians. These situations, despite their intensity, often facilitate psychoanalytic processes. These archaic yearnings lead to other themes—incompletely mourned losses, traumatic experiences, neglectful childhoods, and the like—which then become available for exploration and, at least partially, resolution. Psychoanalysts' love for patients echoes what the ancient Greeks characterized as *agape, philia*, or *storge*. The word *agape* refers to brotherly love. Thomas Aquinas interpreted the Greek word *agape* as willing the good of another. Aristotle, in his Nicomachean ethics, described *philia* as loyalty to friends, family, and community—a love requiring virtue, equality, and familiarity. *Eros*, generally, refers to intimate love. Plato believed that, although *Eros* may be initially felt for a person, contemplation of it brings an appreciation of the beauty within that person. In the *Symposium*, Plato remembers Socrates arguing that *Eros* helps the soul recall knowledge of beauty and spiritual truth. Therefore, for Plato, *Eros* also describes a non-sexual love. The word "Platonic" means "without physical attraction." Lovers and philosophers, Plato believed, sought truth using *Eros*, clearly a major part of the psychoanalysts' task.

Love as safety and reparation

Psychoanalysts' consulting rooms create a type of safety, a privacy, arguably greater than priests' confessionals. They offer sanctuary for the deepest secrets. And yet, self-discovery requires revelations, and revelations require witnesses. Patients have already disclosed as much as they can to themselves. If such auto-confessions sufficed, psychoanalysis need never have emerged as a profession. Carl Rogers[10] believes psychotherapy consists of the opportunity for patients to carefully listen to themselves—like hearing a recording of what they already know. But the process encompasses much more than self-knowledge. Serving almost a maternal function, psychoanalysts create an environment for exploration of not just the self, but of feelings, thoughts, and attitudes toward others, relational patterns, longstanding and repetitive interpersonal schemata, and more.

Even some of the more conservative founders of psychoanalysis wavered on the degree of neutrality required. Freud, for example, particularly as he grew away from conceptualizing psychoanalysis as solely a medical intervention, suggested practitioners serve as "models" or "teachers."[11] Several pioneering psychoanalysts, like Alfred Adler, James Strachey, and Sándor Ferenczi, always worked in a more personal, informal manner. But their ideas were overshadowed by Freud's more conservative emphasis. Fairbairn's psychoanalyst-as-*Exorcist*, discussed earlier and comprising an entire later chapter, implies active, personal participation. He believed clinicians receive, contain, and process "bad objects,"[12] obviously an interpersonal process. Wilfred Bion similarly conceptualized practitioners as "containers"[13] for patients' projections. Later in their careers, both Klein and Fairbairn came to believe that psychoanalytic transformations included patients' internalizing good objects, including their psychoanalysts.

The more interpersonal lines of thinking contributed to the evolution of what many consider a paradigmatic shift: the relational turn, which privileges psychoanalysis' interpersonal elements. Earlier priorities, like the role of drives, were sidelined. The viewpoint became central to Kohut's self-psychology, which introduced the idea of a "transmuting internalization"[14]—meaning the process through which patients introject their psychoanalysts' care for them, leading to a more caring, soothing self-object. He, and similarly oriented psychoanalysts, believe patients cannot help but internalize features of their psychoanalytic relationships. These range from the covert (my psychoanalyst carefully listens to my world) to the overt (he or she clearly cares for me.) These schools of thought share a focus on how psychodynamic psychotherapists' care and attention influence patients.

Nonetheless, psychoanalysts differ in the degree they privilege their personal impact on patients. More conservative psychoanalytic practitioners, who adhere to one-person models of the mind, still emphasize delivering cognitive interpretations to facilitate patients' maturation. They maintain strict professional boundaries. However, even *they* listen extremely carefully. They, too, use their careful attention to dissect and reconfigure patients' harsh superegos. They strive to deconstruct a metaphorical internal parent who, all too often, shouts at the self in angry, judgmental, rejecting tones. These practitioners still rely upon a form of presence.

On the other end of the continuum lie clinicians influenced by the more contemporary models. They tend to be more liberal in interpersonal style. They might share their caring feelings for patients. They may use elements of their own subjectivities as part of the process, and they attend closely to the interpersonal field[15] and other features of two-person (and broader) psychologies. Describing this relational end of the continuum, Schechter writes:

> In more recent years, the relationship *itself* has come to be seen by many psychoanalysts as curative, no longer simply the silent carrier of a more valuable, distinctively psychoanalytic process ... it is precisely the psychoanalyst's ability to have a

relationship with the patient, to experience, process, and contain affective intensity in that relationship, that is of the greatest psychoanalytic value.[16]

Along the same lines, Adam Phillips proclaims:

> I think if people don't care about each other, nothing's going to happen, and if people aren't moved by each other, nothing is going to happen.[17]

Love as danger

I described how Freud compared love in psychotherapeutic relationships to handling explosive substances. And in truth, individuals with primitive personality organizations regress toward seeking literal interpersonal satisfaction. Revealing the influence of Freudian drive theory, Balint specifically identified the wish for "instinctual gratification" in these individuals. Rather than simply behaving seductively, for example, they want to *actually* seduce. These patients deserve just as much presence as others, but psychoanalysts working with them must obviously proceed cautiously. Patients prone toward benign regression tend to have more integrated personality organizations. They wish to be seen or heard authentically, a phenomenon Balint called the regression to recognition.

Regardless of patients' personality organizations, psychoanalysts' maintenance of proper boundaries prevents the much-feared explosions. As noted, sessions should start and end promptly. Other controls are more nuanced. For example, practitioners must be careful if providing sessions late in the day, or early in the morning. These times invite transgressions of traditional taboos. One of my mentors, Jim Grotstein, specifically suggested practitioners avoid providing sessions late on Friday evenings, or at any time during the weekend, because these times signify private, romantic times for psychoanalysts and their spouses or families.

Artistry, love, and psychoanalysis

Whether enhancing or disrupting, the various ways psychoanalysts encounter love in their work highlights the essentially artistic nature of their profession. Maintaining proper boundaries, billing regularly, avoiding late-night sessions, and similar ways psychoanalysts frame their professional relationships barely covers how they deal with loving feelings. Balints' categorization, while informative, is far from infallible. Patients functioning at the level of benign regression can unexpectedly behave in a malignant way; others who typically keep their clinicians at a distance may suddenly feel attracted to them. Some patients, even when regressed into states of weeping, shrieking, or shouting, will receive their psychoanalysts' care simply as acknowledgment. The capacity to make minute-to-minute assessments, to react spontaneously, and to make quick decisions constitute the basic skills required of clinicians. Ringstrom,[18] and I[19] have both written of the ways theatrical analogies arguably best capture the workings of the unconscious mind. Ringstrom writes, "each psychotherapy session represents its own 'stage' in which its participants engage in many 'entrances' and 'exits'" and he emphasizes they not only invite "*dramatic-repetition*" but also create the potential for thematic-altering improvisation.

In sum, psychoanalysts utilize the structured, professional relationship as a transformative vehicle. Years ago, psychoanalytic scholars generated reams of journal articles differentiating between the "real" and the "therapeutic" relationship. In doing so, they promoted a false dichotomy. Psychoanalysts sell a distinct, transformative service. Ideally, they treat their patients with care. Patients need such a loving foundation to feel safe. However, such a loving background does *not*, in and of itself, constitute the transformational service. Remaining focused on facilitating rather than loving is another way of mitigating potential hazards. Further examples from my work with Carlos, Gilda, and Penn illustrate the benefits and risks inherent in how psychoanalysts, in a sense, behave like lovers. They reveal how caring contributes to transformative processes, while equally illustrating how psychoanalysts manage its inevitable emergence.

Carlos

As noted, Carlos abruptly ended our meetings when he felt rejected by my medical leave of absence. The fact that he dismissed me while I was in the hospital, critically ill, mattered naught. The rejection itself validates how significantly love played a role in my relationship with Carlos.

From the get-go, he anticipated a loving relationship. He had constructed an imaginary, idealized image of me—well before we met. The psychologist who referred him similarly idealized me because I had been trained by a mentor of hers. She transferred the veneration to Carlos, who sauntered into my consulting room, expecting to encounter *the great psychoanalyst*. Ultimately, I became as devalued as I had been idealized. Meanwhile, the positive image lingered for months. It likely contributed to Carlos' feeling secure enough to disclose the many horrors to which he had been subjected, and to display the emotional reactions typically accompanying such trauma. He required no warm-up period, exchanges of small talk, or information about my training or experience. During our initial meeting, and as noted earlier, Carlos shared the sadness and anxiety he felt while touring his daughter's school, but he also shared the history of his father's beatings of him, of his leaving the family home when Carlos was five, and of the bullying his two older, half-brothers delivered. Additionally, he felt "invisible" to his cold, distracted, and narcissistic mother. There was no subtlety in the unfolding of the transference.

Never before in my career had I observed such an immediate, powerful paternal transference. As noted earlier, a few months into our work together, Carlos burst into tears, kneeled before me, reached out to hold both of my hands, and asked me to father him. After pausing briefly to ingest the unexpected experience, I tremulously accepted his request. The concreteness of his invitation was strange. After this initial, highly emotional period, Carlos retreated. He often arrived late for sessions; on occasion, he left early, telling me he had pressing business meetings to attend. Overtly, he attempted to regain a less vulnerable position. He seemingly regained control of himself. He asked questions about my life. When I demurred, he changed the subject, misdirecting us away from the denial of his reaction. He bragged about business successes. It was difficult, for a number of months, to bring Carlos' attention to deeper topics.

Perhaps six months into our work together, Carlos and I began the process of dismantling his idealization of me. A phase of more general mourning ensued. He wept at the realization of my clay feet, and the theme was followed by sadness at the painful realization of how every parental figure in his childhood had failed him. He felt I abandoned him by not providing him with the reparative experience he imagined. The idealization, it seemed, had served as an unconscious defense against facing these losses. Carlos thereafter fell into states of intense mourning. When accessing his early experiences, his displays of emotion were remarkable. Quite often, he displayed the emotions of the neglected, abused child he had been. These sessions exemplify the idea of complementary transference.[20] In Carlos' imagination, I represented the depriving parent. He, in turn, re-experienced his archaic feelings of abandonment.

It was precisely during one of these regressed periods that my cardiac valve infection required me to abandon my practice. Interestingly, Carlos worried I developed something serious well before I did. I remember Carlos asking me, on several occasions, if I was ok. I winced when the pain became particularly bad. He asked me if I was getting the best medical care, and offered to help me find various medical specialists. (Here, readers can see another one of Carlos' unconscious maneuvers; by becoming the helper to me, he lessened his vulnerability inherent in the patient role.) After twenty days in the hospital, including open heart surgery to replace an infected aortic valve, my health gradually returned. Two months is a long time for psychoanalytic psychotherapists to vanish. A few weeks before I resumed working, I began contacting patients to schedule appointments. They were uniformly pleased to hear of my recovery. As readers know, all my patients resumed their work with me—except Carlos. Carlos had become immersed in his vulnerability. My medical leave, and its impact on him, happened too quickly for him to defend against it.

Extreme vulnerability lies at the core of individuals with narcissistic personality disorders, and their coping style protects their exquisite vulnerability. Typically, they project it into others. Carlos' habit of arriving late and leaving early, in the few months leading up to my illness, had allowed him to regain some degree of control. He was "never again" going to put himself into the vulnerable position of the patient role. Only after months of establishing a deeper level of trust and connection had he let his guard down again. As we discovered months later, when he eventually returned, Carlos found the experience of my medical crisis overwhelming, and intolerable. It took additional months for him to feel safe again. The reality of the situation mattered naught. As he later explained, he felt angry that his one effort to contact me while I was on medical leave failed. I was too sick to return his call. This, too, proved a severe narcissistic injury to him, resulting in him retreating entirely into his highly defended world.

How does this tale relate to the role of the depth psychotherapist as *Lover*? Precisely because my loving reception for Carlos had invited him to reveal his deeply vulnerable core self. He relinquished his defensive style. In retrospect, the transformative power of the first season of our work is primarily attributable to my role as *Lover*. Emboldened by our initial year of work together, Carlos had opened up. Carlos' awareness of the seemingly benign back condition, suddenly resulting in hospitalization for a more serious condition, contributed to Carlos' shock. By analogy, his *Lover*, with whom he experienced the most intimate closeness of his entire life, suddenly left him. Worse, he then failed in a promise to return his call. Still worse, he nearly died. It took an entire second season, and nearly a year, for Carlos to even begin to regain the kind of trust he had in me that first season of our work together.

Gilda

My assuming the role of *Lover* in my work with Gilda demonstrates how Balints' idea of a malignant regression, combined with my clumsiness, created an almost literal perversion. The first period of my work with her, before anonymous assailants attacked her after her firm's holiday party, illustrates how practitioners behave like *Lovers* while maintaining proper boundaries. My caring presence invited Gilda into an exposed, intimate openness. My use of the word "clumsy" likely represents my own shame at how I later lost my way. Imagine working in any professional role, opening the waiting room door, and seeing a remarkably attractive woman. My enchantment exponentially expanded within a few minutes of actually encountering her—her brilliance, the prosody of her speech, and the way her mouth moved when she talked. She even gestured with grace. I struggled to contain my reaction to her, mentally retrieving the rules of engagement when feeling so positively toward a new patient.

I succeeded, at least during the first two years, in behaving professionally. I carefully listened to her history, following its many winding, tortuous turns. Metaphorically, I walked by her side. I witnessed her grief as she processed the termination with her prior depth psychotherapist, received the updates on his deteriorating health, and learned the details of his death. I sat quietly with her when she wept. Only after days and weeks of empathic listening, I helped her parse the reaction to his death—separating out true grief from her propensity to believe she had somehow contributed. Occasionally distracted by vivid romantic and sexual fantasies about her, I nonetheless succeeded in providing the various behaviors comprising presence. I felt sympathetic. I cared for her. My more dangerous feelings remained in bounds. In all likelihood, she sensed my affection and care and, as already suggested, it created the safe, welcoming, womb-like environment patients need.

Before delving into how I lost my way with Gilda—for the year following her injury—I scroll back in to review how transference-countertransference configurations can be much more complicated than some of the simplified examples I have presented. My initial reaction to Gilda speaks many truths about *me*—need states, aesthetic preferences, themes problematic and not. My own mother had treated me much like Carlos' had, depriving me of the kind of loving attention that builds a solid sense of self. It left me hungry for female attention. Months later, Gilda perhaps played into my attraction. But it is important to emphasize how much of that original reaction concerns my psychodynamics, not hers.

As we became better acquainted, we both played a role in the unfolding of the transference–countertransference configuration. Gilda had been terrifically abandoned by both of her parents. Difficult to separate out the chicken from the egg, she either pulled for, or I offered, the rescue she desperately desired. I have already repeatedly shared my own weakness, of sorts, toward assuming the role of the rescuer. This dynamic represented one of the primary ways the transference and countertransference developed between us. A secondary pattern developed, and deserves separate consideration because of its accelerating nature. The more Gilda yearned for my rescue or, alternatively, the more I strived to do so, the more we both regressed. She became almost a raw, extremely needy baby; I fell deeply into the role of the omnipotent parent, required to soothe her every need. Common to working with acutely traumatized adults, I experienced other typical countertransference reactions, including a propensity to feel overwhelmed by her pain and to experience abject feelings of helplessness and powerlessness.

I have long struggled against feelings of powerlessness, and I feel particularly sensitive to them. Therefore, between the pull to rescue Gilda, and the normal powerlessness one experiences when working with traumatized patients, the work became almost unbearable for me. I could neither rescue Gilda from her childhood pain nor could I salve her post-traumatic distress. At various times during the period after she was attacked, I found myself becoming sleepy during sessions. Never before had meetings with her elicited such drowsiness. In retrospect, I consider it an unconscious way to avoid my own discomfort. My own empathic experiencing of Gilda's pain was intense.

In the prior chapter, I described the various ways I brought the perverse and destructive psychoanalytic process with Gilda back into a proper and workable frame. Most relevant to this chapter is how I transitioned back into the role of *Lover* in its proper psychoanalytic sense. It illustrates the fragile balance required, session to session, to utilize the *Lover* role to its maximal potential. Several of my behaviors crossed the line into behaving *literally* like a lover, rather than assuming the social role in an authentic but bounded way. For example, I began sharing the depth of my concern for her. I told her how powerless I felt, particularly during those months she fell into the psychogenic fugue states. When the attack and subsequent disability drained her financial reserves, I engaged in a dual relationship with Gilda by employing her. I broke traditional boundaries by reaching out to her orthopedic surgeon, her lawyers, and her daughter. I took the "mutual recognition"[21] espoused by Jessica Benjamin to its logical, if aberrant, extreme. I strayed well beyond optimal provision into behaving like a real other or, worse, like a real lover. I became her peer, and also her employer.

The road back to establishing a proper psychoanalytic frame was as could be expected—rocky and perilous. Gilda, understandably and legitimately, became enraged at me. Here, again, the errors of scholars separating the therapeutic from the real relationship become obvious. The two social roles become blurred, in every case, but in this case I clearly overstepped. As I pulled back, Gilda had every reason to feel anger. Her subsequent perception of me as in retreat was neither symbolic nor imagined. I actually pulled away. I felt I had to. On the level of the transference–countertransference, my withdrawal also triggered deeper, archaic unconscious wounds in Gilda. I became the mother who called her ugly and stupid, and who also withdrew from her. Because I had moved too close, I became the sexual abuser. My excessive self-disclosures, over-involvement, and engaging her as analyst, employer, and friend were experienced by Gilda as violating. The resultant fury at me represented a panoply of real reactions to me combined with unresolved rage at the prior historical violations, namely the childhood molestation, the adolescent sexual assault, and the more recent attack.

Yet another irony, my properly resuming the role of the *Lover* proved a crucial part in my returning our relationship back to its proper bounds. It contained her rage as I returned to behaving in a normal, professional manner. I listened carefully, avoiding defensive reactions. I empathized, limited my self-disclosures, and stopped talking to collateral parties. I metaphorically gritted my teeth while experiencing those difficult emotions for me—helplessness, powerlessness, as well as an overwhelming feeling of empathy for her post-traumatic pain. My ability—amplified by meetings with a more senior colleague who provided me with some degree of objectivity—to remain in the *Lover* role during this transition period proved crucial. Had I reacted to her fury with my own anger, or had I withdrawn excessively like her mother had, Gilda would never have made her way back to a middle zone of relating with me. The role of *Lover*, even though, admittedly, I enacted it too literally during the middle period, may well have been most crucial in helping Gilda recover from not only the childhood wounds we had opened up in our work together, but also to recover from the injuries I myself inflicted upon her.

Penn

With Penn, the role of *Lover* played out much less dramatically than with Carlos or with Gilda. It provided the same sense of safety offered to the other two patients. In Penn's case, however, the role uniquely served to dissolve his powerful intellectual defenses. Also, it invited me to gently explore, and then more aggressively confront, the way he avoided deeper encounters through his habitual tardiness. Together, we discovered that Penn's consistently running late served as a means of avoiding vulnerability. (Interestingly, Carlos' tardiness served the same function, but it only appeared after he had become vulnerable; Penn ran late from the start.) Consulting depth psychotherapists puts patients in vulnerable positions no matter what, but for Penn, leaning into the chronic, underlying anxiety—plaguing him for as long as he could remember— was nearly intolerable. He ran late in all areas of his life, resulting in his chronically "feeling rushed." Ironically, the solution created the same problem it intended to solve—anxiety. Rather than understanding and addressing the archaic causes of his nervousness, he instead became unconsciously engaged in tricking himself. On a conscious level, he attributed his anxiety to the reality of his "always rushing." He tended to become quiet in other situations when he felt anxious, and he struggled to begin sessions (which I considered a form of resistance). He'd often start with, "I cannot think of anything to say today."

Few psychoanalytic interpretations have the kind of immediate impact when I suggested the connection between his "driven" lifestyle, his tardiness with me, his initial withdrawal during sessions, and the underlying anxiety. Penn had an "aha" moment. Within a week, he began attending sessions on time. Penn began viewing his prompt arrivals as an opportunity to investigate his anxiety. Ironically, he thereafter *strived* to arrive early. Sometimes, I saw the annunciator light come on as much as 5 or 10 minutes before our start time. According to Penn, he'd sit in the waiting room, set his cell phone aside, avoid reading magazines, and simply reflect on how he felt. The reception of the insight, and the resultant behavioral change, could only have occurred in an environment in which he felt emotionally supported.

Regarding his specific sensitivities, Penn's anxiety represented underlying and deep feelings of inadequacy that drive his compulsive need to work. The compensatory style served two distinct functions: It allowed him to channel anxiety into activities—evaluating patients, performing surgeries, studying, and writing; it also bolstered his sense of competence. Penn's behavior validates one of Thomas Szasz' quips: Patients consult depth psychotherapists because of solutions, not problems. [22] Their solutions have become their problem. Penn's lifestyle perfectly validates Szasz' point. His work not only provided a conduit for his anxiety; it also justified it. At the same time, it salved the inadequacy. He "fooled" himself, to use his own words, "feeling like an important man, always on the run." Penn's working life eclipsed most other aspects of his life: He rarely participated in any non-work-related recreational activities, he lacked intimate friendships, he spent little time with his wife or children, and he rarely enjoyed free, spontaneous, fun-filled moments. Put another way, his life became dull. While the compulsive overwork was the currency he paid for anxiety relief, it also created a psychological dreariness.

Penn learned of these explanations mostly through my functioning as a *Critic*. Given his relative maturity, the *Exorcist* function played a lesser role in our work than it did with either of the other two patients. However, and returning to the tardiness issue, here was an area in which some projective identification occurred. While waiting for him, I was placed in the vulnerable position. I'd keep my eye on my annunciator light, listen for sounds in the waiting room, or check my voicemail messages. I could not start a significant project, like writing a report or calling a colleague, because of the limbo state. I experienced, through projective identification, a variety of *his* vulnerability. The experience represents one of the ways my role as *Exorcist* helped Penn. By experiencing the projection, processing it, and then later presenting it to him, he could assume the feeling he had projected into me. It is an excellent example of how an experience, projected out, can come to be reintegrated by patients in psychodynamic psychotherapy.

However, and again, such means of engagement *only* work when layered upon the foundational level of psychoanalysts' emotional presence or, to continue with the metaphor, in their underlying role as *Lover*. The roles of *Exorcist* and *Critic* proceed in relatively straightforward ways, and I will explain them in depth in the coming chapters. Clinicians may interpret projective processes, as just illustrated. At other times, they directly confront them. These are, in a sense, variations of education. Like critics giving notes to novelists, playwrights, or artists, depth psychotherapists observe and then describe their observations of the repetition compulsion, dreams, or other manifestations of the unconscious emerging in the work. They tend to focus on transference and countertransference themes because they occur in real time during actual sessions. However, when it comes to the always emotionally laden process of depth psychotherapy, the *Lover* role works in somewhat more mysterious ways.

The simple, caring reception of patients' emotional experiences contributes to the repairing of previously traumatic experiences. With Penn, specifically, my assuming the role of *Lover* mimicked the way a plastic surgeon might repair an unsightly, infected scar. Surgeons re-open the poorly healed wound, treat the infection, debride scar tissue, and then carefully re-suture the area. Invariably, patients, when healed, are left with a smaller scar. In like manner, psychoanalysts uncover any number of psychic injuries, whether from early childhood or adult-onset trauma, observe the wounds in partnership with their patients, and then address and resolve the related deficits or conflicts in a way reducing, but rarely eliminating, the emotional scarring.

Over time, and only because of the consistently caring attitude I showed him, Penn began—slowly, tenuously, gradually—to *feel* the anxiety, and the sense of inadequacy underlying it. As noted, he deliberately experienced them prior to our sessions while waiting. The combination of my caring, and his receptivity, created an emotionally intimate relationship between us. He began slowing down. Not only did he literally talk less rapidly, but his speeding through sessions, much like he rushed through life, decreased. Perhaps a year into our work, an entirely new pattern developed between the two of us. I would greet Penn warmly in the waiting room, escort him into my consulting room, and then sit quietly, allowing silence to fill the space of the room. I deliberately waited for Penn to start speaking. He stopped his initial tendency to begin by reporting he had "nothing to discuss." He expressed his thoughts and feelings wandering in a variety of directions.

Once our encounters slowed down, Penn became more overtly emotional. Sometimes, his eyes filled with tears as he remembered what he called "the terrors." The stories of his childhood experience became more elaborate. One of his earliest memories, for example, involved playing with toy trucks on a cold, Spanish-tiled floor while his mother angrily washed the dishes in the nearby kitchen. He remembered, viscerally, how fearful he felt. He recalled sharpening his ears for the sound of the garage door openings, signaling the return of his father from work. For the first fourteen years of his life, his father served a maternal function. Penn ran into his arms when his father entered the house. He represented comfort to him, whereas his mother represented rage.

Such archaic early childhood scenes often serve an organizing function for patients. They represent mathematical fractals for their lives, templates influencing their perceptions of the world. Penn's frightening scene, fearing his mother and awaiting his father, illustrates such a pattern. Penn, playing alone on a cold tile floor, feared an outburst from his angry, agitated mother. He looked forward to the warmth of his father's return. However, the anticipated respite only partially quelled his discomfort. We figured, based on other memories recovered by Penn over the years, that his mother resented parenting. She felt irritated, ungratified, and distracted. His home environment was anything but loving and supportive. The early memory created a lasting impression, later offering hints about Penn's complex relationship with his father.

After months of psychotherapy sessions, Penn fell into still deeper states of emotion. There were periods in which he wept off and on for weeks at a time, mourning the absence of a loving mother. Much later, we discovered what we, together, called a "double abandonment." In the midst of the usual teenage angst, when Penn was fourteen or fifteen, he began to express overt anger at his mother. Discussed at greater length in the chapter on the *Critic*, Penn's father faced an implacable problem: Does he honor the concerns of his son, potentially leading to a disruption in his marriage? Or does he retreat? Unfortunately for Penn, his father chose to withdraw from him. During sessions following this understanding, Penn faced the ambivalence he felt toward his father. In some ways, his father saved him, offering him crucial support. But his capacity for empathy was limited, and the overt withdrawal proved injurious. Emotions other than sadness and mourning emerged. Penn became infuriated at times, particularly at what he called "my father's choice to retreat." In retrospect, these highly emotional encounters demonstrate the process of Penn working through childhood trauma. His simply reliving memories, with their associated emotionality, fomented psychic transformation. These processes could only evolve in the presence of the caring other, namely me behaving as a variety of *Lover*. One can easily understand how patients become cognitively aware of the psychodynamics of a repetitive pattern, a dream, or transference configurations. The intricacies of working through trauma, unmet needs states, or conflicts—in the presence of a stable, caring other—create an emotional transformation more difficult to describe. In the final analysis, the role of *Lover* facilitates transformation more significantly than purely cognitive understanding allows.

Transference, countertransference, and the *Lover*

Between the regularity of the meeting times, the framing of the professional relationships, and the minimally benign interest paid to patients by practitioners, patients cannot help but regress into a transferential relationship with their clinicians. As Lacan views it, patients perceive psychoanalysts as "subjects presumed to know."[23] Patients react to the inherent power differential along a continuum ranging from slavish submission to tyrannical dominance. Some patients perceive their depth psychotherapists as loving, protective mothers, fathers, or uncles; others view them as punishing, depriving authority figures. These themes characterize transference phenomena, and the psychoanalyst-as-*Lover* contributes to these reactions. Countertransference functions in much the same way. Certainly, psychoanalytic clinicians begin working with patients by showing interest, caring, respect, and other features of presence. Over time, however, these attitudes morph.

Some clinicians become overly worried, erotically aroused, or otherwise positively inclined toward patients. Others may develop negative feelings like envy, aggression, and even hatred. Emotional reactions to patients, running parallel to their transference themes, constitute the countertransference. Depth psychotherapy requires of its practitioners an always-imperfect capacity for introspection. They hopefully consider their feelings for patients might reflect their own personal world, a projection by patients, a combination, or even a unique, complex emotional reaction emerging from that psychoanalytic couple. In conclusion, then, the role of *Lover* facilitates all features of psychodynamic psychotherapy. Inevitably, it also invites projection. Such projective processes require depth psychotherapists to assume an entirely different role, one I explore in detail next, namely the role of the *Exorcist*.

Notes

1. Geertz, C. (2000). *Local knowledge: Further Essays in Interpretive Anthropology*. New York, NY: Basic Books, p. 79.

2. Freud, S. (1915). Observations on transference-love (further recommendations on the technique of psycho-analysis III). *The Standard Edition of the Complete Psychological Works of Sigmund Freud, Volume XII (1911–1913): The Case of Schreber, Papers on Technique and Other Works*. London: Hogarth Press, London: Hogarth Press, pp. 157–171.

3. Freud, S. (1910). "Wild" psycho-analysis. *The Standard Edition of the Complete Psychological Works of Sigmund Freud, Volume XI (1910): Five Lectures on Psycho-Analysis, Leonardo da Vinci and Other Works*. London: Hogarth Press, pp. 219–228.

4. Freud, S. (1915). Observations on transference-love (further recommendations on the technique of psycho-analysis III). *The Standard Edition of the Complete Psychological Works of Sigmund Freud, Volume XII (1911–1913): The Case of Schreber, Papers on Technique and Other Works*. London: Hogarth Press, London: Hogarth Press, pp. 157–171, p. 165.

5. Ibid., p. 170.

6. Ibid., p. 170.

7. Ibid., pp. 170–171.

8. Poland, W.S. (2000). The analyst's witnessing and otherness. *Journal of the American Psychoanalytic Association*, 48: 17–34.

9. Bowlby, J. (1980). *Attachment: Attachment and Loss* (Vol. 1). New York, NY: Basic Books; Bowlby, J. (1980). *Separation: Anxiety and Anger* (Vol. 2). New York, NY: Basic Books; Bowlby, J. (1980). *Loss: Sadness and Depression* (Vol. 3). New York, NY: Basic Books; Ainsworth, M.D. (1982). Attachment: Retrospect and prospect. In C.M. Parkes & J. Stevenson-Hinde (Eds.), *The Place of Attachment in Human Behavior*. London: Tavistock; Main, M. (2000). The organized categories of infant, child, and adult attachment. *Journal of the American Psychoanalytic Association*, 48, 1055–1095.

10. Rogers, C. (1961). *On Becoming a Person—A Psychotherapist's View of Psychotherapy*. New York, NY: Houghton Mifflin.

11. Freud, S. (1937). Analysis terminable and interminable. *International Journal of Psycho-Analysis*, 18: 373–405.

12. Fairbairn, W.R.D. (1952). *Psychoanalytic Studies of the Personality*. London: Tavistock.

13. Bion, W.R. (1962). *Learning from Experience*. London: Tavistock, p. 90.

14. Kohut, H. (1984). *How Does Analysis Cure?* Chicago, IL: University of Chicago Press.

15. Baranger, M., & Baranger, W. (2009). Spiral process and the dynamic field. In L.G. Fiorini (Eds.), *The Work of Confluence: Listening and Interpreting in the Psychoanalytic Field*. London: Karnac, pp. 45–61. (Original work published in 1979.)

16. Schechter, K. (2014). *Illusions of a Future: Psychoanalysis and the Biopolitics of Desire*. Durham, NC: Duke University Press, p. 2.

17. Choder-Goldman, J. (2014). An interview with Adam Phillips. *Psychoanalytic Perspectives*, 11(3): 334–347, p. 342.

18. Ringstrom, P. (2018). Three dimensional field theory: dramatization and improvisation in a psychoanalytic theory of change. *Psychoanalytic Dialogues*, 28: 379–396. Doi.org/10.1080/1048 1885.2018.1482128, pp. 389 and 395.

19. Karbelnig, A. (2020). The theater of the unconscious mind. *Psychoanalytic Psychology*, 37(4), 273–281.

20. Racker, H. (1982). *Transference and Countertransference*. London: Routledge.

21. Benjamin, J. (1988). *The Bonds of Love: Psychoanalysis, Feminism, and the Problem of Domination*. New York, NY: Random House.

22. Szasz, T. (1988). *The Ethics of Psychoanalysis*. Syracuse, NY: The Syracuse University Press.

23. Lacan, J. (1998). *The Seminar of Jacques Lacan, Book XI: The Four Fundamental Concepts of Psychoanalysis*. J. Miller (Ed.) & A. Sheridan (Trans.). New York, NY: Norton, p. 232. (Original work published in 1973.)

CHAPTER 7

The *Exorcist*

On the two occasions I taught psychodynamic psychotherapy to students in China, I saw them struggling mightily with the concept of an exorcism. Their culture is steeped in Taoism and Buddhism—religious philosophies lacking the kinds of exorcisms as understood in the West. I endeavored to teach them about it using projective identification. They understood such primitive defense mechanisms without difficulty, but when switching to exorcism as a metaphor, they seemed confused. I hope the metaphor makes sense to you readers.

The word "exorcism," derived from the ancient Greek *exorkismos*, means binding by an oath. In Christianity, specifically, exorcism refers to casting out demons. The priest performing the exorcism, graced with special powers or skills, typically invokes God, Jesus, or different angels or archangels to intervene. Catholic clergy distinguish between formal exorcisms, which can only be conducted by a priest, and "prayers of deliverance," which anyone can conduct. Formal exorcisms proceed by swearing an oath, performing an elaborate ritual, and commanding the demons to depart. The concept of exorcism exists in other religious traditions as well. For example, one of the four Vedas—the holy books of the Hindus—the Atharva Veda, contains the secrets of exorcism. Some Islamic Mullahs perform exorcisms, a practice called *ruqya*. It is used to repair the damage caused by black magic or *sihr*. Exorcisms are performed within the Jewish tradition, typically by Rabbis trained in Kabbalah. Exorcisms also occur in Taoism, a piece of historical trivia likely left out of Chinese students' contemporary education. Within Taoism, a person might become possessed by disturbing a ghost who seeks revenge. The exorcist calms the disturbance.

In his book *Madness and Civilization*, Foucault[1] traces how the medical profession, and its allies, took over responsibility for persons previously attended to by the Church during the Enlightenment. Christian churches, in particular, began caring for the mentally ill. In parallel fashion, people who were thought to be possessed by demons were sent to medical professionals rather than clergy. Of course, these practitioners did not formally offer exorcisms. Or did they? Freud made no direct references to exorcism himself, although he published a 1923 paper titled "A seventeenth-century demonological neurosis."[2] Object relations theories spawned the possibility of analogies to exorcisms. These models invited theorists to think of ways persons split their internal worlds, and project part of them out, eliciting phenomena looking much like demonic possessions. I cited Fairbairn's famous quotation earlier, but it begs for a paraphrased review. Using the idea of the True Mass as consciousness, and the Black Mass as the unconscious mind, Fairbairn notes how psychotherapists replace exorcists. They concern themselves not only with forgiving sins, but with casting out devils (meaning the bad objects in patients' internal dramas).

What does Fairbairn mean? He suggests that, while patients describe their conscious experiences during sessions, they unconsciously enact a different type of internal drama. Depth psychotherapists are primarily concerned, of course, with what occurs in the crypt. They may disagree about many elements of the theory of mind and practice, but all psychoanalysts agree that their work is concerned primarily with bringing disavowed, hidden, or unconscious parts of human subjectivity into the conscious domain. By working with their patients' projections, often accompanied by sadness, anger, loss, or other intense emotional experiences, depth psychotherapists indeed behave like exorcists. Their ritual takes place within the sanctity of the consulting room; their authority resides in their social role, and; their secular prayers consist of the psychoanalytic process itself.

Projective identification and demonic possession

The concept of projective identification is one of the most difficult ideas to understand regarding depth psychotherapy. Risking repetitiveness, I will explain it several times because of its inherent difficulty. Technically, the word *projection* is encompassed by the phrase, *projective identification*. That latter word, identification, denotes how projections occur when persons *identify* them. Pure projection rarely occurs. For example, a friend of mine once walked hurriedly toward a subway in Paris. She followed streams of people headed in the same direction. Suddenly, a woman walking in front of her spun around and shouted, "Stop following me!" Here, that rare, pure form of projection occurred. My friend had no reason to think the woman in front of her thought she was being followed. And, of course, my friend was *not* actually following the woman. If you are feeling your friend's anger projected into you, you only experience it if you *identify* with that feeling. In brief, you introject it, and then you identify with, or experience, it.

Projective identification occurs on interpersonal as well as intrapsychic levels. Interpersonal projective identification occurs when a projection is hurled by party A, received by party B, and party B reacts. I just offered one example. Here is another: Consider persons exhibiting passive-aggressive behavior. These individuals harbor anger toward others, but have difficulty directly expressing it. If angry at their supervisor at work, for example, they might be late, fail to complete assignments, speak in a whiny voice tone, or otherwise express their irritation *indirectly*. These persons typically cause those around them to feel angry. The tardiness, incomplete assignments, and whininess elicit anger in their supervisors—a hopefully clear illustration of projective identification. Through subtle, unconscious, nonverbal behaviors, passive-aggressive individuals project their anger into others.

Depending on their personal preference and theoretical orientation, some psychoanalysts simply explain such passive-aggressive tendencies to their patients. Others who are more relationally oriented may disclose how the patient's behavior elicits angry feelings in them. In any event, when their patients manifest passive aggression, depth psychotherapists will almost always feel the anger themselves. Next, they describe the process to their patients, including how it fits in with new or already established themes in their lives. Other emotional states can be projected out in unconscious ways. Persons struggling with significant sadness may elicit sad feelings in those around them; those struggling with significant anxiety, guilt, shame, grief, or other strong emotional states will similarly communicate them interpersonally.

Projective identification may involve processes other than emotions. Individuals may project other types of mental content or, even specific mental functioning. Oppositional adolescents, for example, typically elicit in their parents a desire to take some form of action for them. These teenagers project *agency*. Along the same lines, certain passive patients, who may ask their depth psychotherapists for specific direction, may also project agency. They might ask, "Do you think I should break up with my girlfriend?" They might ask for guidance about a job, a friend, or another area of their lives. In these instances, practitioners typically feel pulled to act on behalf of the patient—the felt-invitation representing a form of projective identification. Since the psychodynamic psychotherapies are also united in their devotion to empowering patients or, in other words, to enhancing their sense of control or agency over their own lives, they routinely process such projective identification processes. The more direct persons' expressions of anger, the more autonomy they have.

Arguably the *most* difficult psychoanalytic concept to explain is the idea of *intrapsychic* projective identification. If projective identification is like moving mental content between different rooms in a house, then it also refers to moving these parts around within an individual mind. An intolerable level of anger, for example, can be unconsciously transferred from the ego to the superego, to use the Freudian metaphors. Such a person will then experience a *more* punishing version of the superego. A harsher, angrier attitude toward the self may result. Intrapsychic projective identification is, obviously, a clear example of a one-person model of mind.

In real life, interpersonal and intrapsychic projective identification operate in consonance with one another. Psychoanalyst James Grotstein named such a process "the dual mode of psychological functioning."

We exist simultaneously under the control of our internal dramas as well as the interpersonal, social field. Previously, I proposed the philosophy of perspectivism as a foundational philosophy. It applies when integrating these different models of projective identification. The one-person (intrapsychic) and two-person (interpersonal) psychologies offer different perspectives on projective identification. Although dissection proves useful for explaining these processes, they occur in such an intertwined manner that separating them only works in the abstract.

Consider persons who unconsciously intrapsychically transfer excessive rage from the ego to the superego, like I just mentioned. Internally, they typically end up as highly self-critical persons. Externally, they view others through the same filter: They may expect criticism from others they encounter; alternatively, they may project their ego onto others and tend to behave in a critical, judgmental way toward them. The internal and external worlds exist in a dynamic balance with each other, a concept captured, at least in part, by Robert Stolorow's phrase, "dynamic intersubjective systems."[3] We swim in an interpersonal soup, controlled in part by our individual organismic drives. These, in turn, come under the influence of interpersonal and cultural forces, and so on, *ad infinitum*. The person with the harsh superego who, subjected to harsh criticism from a supervisor a few hours after learning his wife left him, might well erupt into a state of extreme rage. He could become violent. Alternatively, he might fall to pieces, weeping uncontrollably and writhing on the street corner until paramedics arrive and transfer him to a psychiatric facility. Observers might think a devil took possession of him. If he lived in the Middle Ages, others almost certainly would have considered him possessed.

Projective identification and defense mechanisms

In the early days of psychoanalysis, practitioners prepared themselves to encounter resistance from patients. They worked aggressively to break through the repression barrier, releasing affect-laden memories intended to facilitate change in patients. Lacan believes patients become accustomed to, and even love, their symptoms. These viewpoints suggest psychoanalysts should distrust their patients, think them lying, hiding, and subverting. Orange calls such an attitude the "hermeneutics of suspicion" rather than the "hermeneutics of trust."[4] Ringstrom believes patients fear repeating their problematic repetitive patterns as much as they fear *not* repeating them. He interprets resistance in a new and more humanistic light. In other words, we all resist change. Resistance no longer signifies psychopathology; it signifies normalcy. Since the relational turn, depth psychotherapists expect patients to resist change.

Psychoanalysts promote regression—even if only by virtue of their social role. As noted in the last chapter, their caring presence, and even the den-like furnishings of their offices, unwittingly invite confessions, the sharing of intimate thoughts and feelings, and other oft-hidden information. Both parties participate in searching for signs of the unconscious mind, and here is where the concept of defense mechanisms are important. The sanctuary-like environment tends to relax patients' usual defensive styles. Nonetheless, such protective mechanisms stand at-the-ready, covering up uncomfortable conflicts or need states or other experiences felt to be (unconsciously) too shameful or distressing to discuss.

The post-Freudians, including most contemporary psychoanalysts, still identify projective identification and splitting as the most primitive forms of defense mechanisms. They might call them by different names, but the phenomena associated with these words is well understood. Splitting organizes their world in the simplest manner possible. Hurtful people, objects, or any source of discomfort are viewed as bad; feelings of love, wholeness, or tranquility are considered good. In parallel, infants rely heavily on projective identification. I presented the concept several times, and here is yet another review from a new angle: Projective identification is a primal means of communication. Most caregivers learn, quickly, the unique cries of their babies: Some indicate hunger, others fatigue, and still others a need for a diaper change. Such nonverbal communication represents normal projective identification. Babies cannot speak; ergo, they use nonverbal ways of communicating. The splitting or projective identification in infancy does not imply psychopathology; it is a normal developmental stage, which Melanie Klein called the paranoid–schizoid position.[5] Part of the transition out of the stage occurs when parents advise their children to "use your words." The development of language enhances the ability to utilize more mature defensive mechanisms, and, thereafter, splitting and projective identification become marginalized.

Meanwhile, projective identification, like splitting, helps infants cope with their worlds. The way they project out any number of uncomfortable emotions, and how their caregivers identify and respond to them, allows babies to manage their lives. It promotes development as they internalize caregiver reactions, project out more of their feelings and behaviors and so on in an ongoing, cyclic manner. Splitting creates the qualitative split by organizing the world into categories of good and bad; projective identification creates a geographical split by moving mental content around internally or interpersonally. I described these concepts earlier, but they bear review because of their key role in understanding how psychoanalysts assume the *Exorcist* role.

Although mature persons utilize primitive defense mechanisms less frequently, they still use them in extreme situations. For example, if two masked individuals suddenly smashed through the window in the room in which you are quietly reading this book, and pointed machine guns at you, you would immediately regress into the paranoid–schizoid position. Your world view would become dominated by splitting and projective identification. You would identify as good, and the intruders as bad. You would lose your capacity for empathy. These processes would all occur unconsciously, and literally within nanoseconds. You would not wonder about the assailants' abusive childhood experience, or whether their desperate economic situations led them to take such drastic action. Instead, you would project your black-and-white view of the world onto them. They are bad; you are good. You concern yourself with safety, evasion, begging, pleading, or using a weapon for protection. The paranoid–schizoid position is pre-moral for just this reason. Splitting and projective identification are survival-oriented, primitive defense mechanisms. Of course, much more benign examples of the use of splitting and projective identification exist in typical life. I offer this only as but one extreme example.

Patients often project more mature affects onto their depth psychotherapists. They may assume their clinicians will show them the loving attention of a good parent. Or they may expect a more mature form of a critic, or even just a benign observer of their lives. When considering the depth psychotherapists' role as *Exorcist*, however, primitive mental processes are inevitably involved. The situations in which patients think you hate them, fall hopelessly in love with you, or impulsively leave a session while shouting, "You are awful; I will never return," bring demonic analogies to mind.

Some believe the processing of projective identification is the heart of all depth psychotherapeutic work. Wilfred Bion, for example, wrote extensively about how psychoanalytic clinicians process patients' projective identifications—even though he never used the word "exorcism" specifically. He referred to primitive projections as "alpha elements." Bion believes psychoanalysts spend most of their time absorbing, digesting, and converting these projections into "beta elements."[6] He thinks psychoanalysts serve as "containers" for these projections. Through processes like confrontation, interpretation, clarifying feelings, and similar interventional methods, psychoanalysts create secular exorcisms. At the end of a course of successful depth psychotherapy, patients ideally become more aware of unconsciously harbored feelings of anger toward their father, or yearning for love from their mother, or competitiveness with a sibling of which they were previously unaware. Any number of emotions, traumatic childhood scenarios, or behaviors eventually enter the subjectivities of psychoanalytic practitioners who, in turn, gradually introduce them back to their patients. When dramatic, the process looks much like exorcisms, which invites me to illustrate the analogy using examples from my work with Carlos, Gilda, and Penn.

Carlos

Carlos resides, developmentally, primarily in the paranoid–schizoid position. When he abruptly ended his depth psychotherapy immediately after I became ill, he was projecting out his vulnerability. A frightened, deeply insecure little boy inside, Carlos found my transformation into being more vulnerable than him intolerable. Using Fairbairn's analogy, Carlos felt concern for me on the level of True Mass. He worried about my sudden exit; he was hurt I failed to make my appointment with him on the day of my hospitalization or return his phone call while there. On the level of the Black Mass, my illness was nothing less than catastrophic. His idealization of himself in twinship transference with me abruptly collapsed. Carlos likely felt, unconsciously, abandoned, alone, and hopeless. He dealt with the situation, unconsciously, by reversing roles with me.

Notice how the offer he made to me, including taking me to dinner or otherwise assuming a normal social role, involved removing him from a vulnerable position. They allowed for him to remain invulnerable, to initiate social contact and pay for it. I would assume the role of his guest or invitee. I felt deeply hurt by Carlos when I first heard those voicemails from him, reacting with guilt and shame. Had I erred in some way? Fairly quickly, however, I realized his verbalizations as forms of projective identification. Notice how the feelings I just described mirror, quite accurately, emotions he had expressed in our first season. While listening to his voicemail messages, I felt possessed. As I regained my strength, and communicated by phone and email with Carlos, I felt more confident in my ability to use my emotional reactions to help him.

Patients like Carlos tend to elicit extremely uncomfortable feelings in psychodynamic psychotherapists. It requires time and experience to learn to channel the hurt, anger, sadness, or other intense affects they experience into facilitating transformational experiences for them. They learn to respond rather than react to such provocations. Once Carlos resumed weekly sessions, and, later, twice-weekly ones—on conditions set by him—I often served in the role of *Exorcist*. For example, I interpreted the role reversal and the projection of his vulnerability that occurred after I was hospitalized. Of course, the exploration of its historical origins occurred while assuming the role of *Critic*—but we'll discuss that in the next chapter. Meanwhile, Carlos seemed accepting of the *Lover*, the *Exorcist*, and the *Critic* for about as long as he could tolerate it, which was around a year.

After exiting the second season, another striking possession episode happened. Carlos relinquished his use of tranquilizing drugs and alcohol during those months after he stopped coming in. This, of course, was an extremely positive development. He proudly shared his sobriety as soon as our meetings resumed. However, and as a replacement behavior, Carlos became compulsively involved in bodybuilding. He attended Gold's Gym on a daily basis. He became personally acquainted with Arnold Schwarzenegger, who went to the same gym every day. One day, while describing his muscle-enhancing work, Carlos abruptly stood up. Before I realized what was occurring, he took off his sweatshirt and his sweatpants. He stood wearing only his bikini-style underwear bottoms. Anticipating some intervention, Carlos ran to the other side of my consulting room. He flexed his arm and leg muscles, just like you would imagine, assuming typical bodybuilding postures. I feared he would remove his underpants. Fortunately for both of us, he kept them on. He asked me to observe his various muscle groups he pointed out as he moved from one stance to another. I did. I was transfixed.

Here, again, Carlos' behavior essentially demanded I behave as *Exorcist*. The needy-boy-child within him begged for attention. I could not help but feel, quite literally, like the admiring parental figure for which he yearned. I could have reacted with anger; I could have reacted with negative judgment. Instead, I felt, and then expressed, my true admiration for the way his body glistened. He had intentionally lost weight. He looked like a young Schwarzenegger. The episode exemplifies the dual operations of the internal and external worlds. On an intrapsychic level, Carlos had split his mind into parts. He became entirely identified with the small, insecure child looking for admiration; interpersonally, Carlos elicited the nonverbal interaction just described, and which he desperately desired.

Before switching over to *Critic*, I remained the *Exorcist* who took on the demon in the patient. Rather than a demon, though, the approving, admiring, loving other, whom he yearns for every day of his life, took complete possession of me. In fact, I was speechless for the first few seconds. It was only after that brief period that I shared my admiration. At no point did I interpret the behavior—at least for the rest of *that* session. He disrobed shortly before our time was up. I only had time to feel the nearly overwhelming reactions of fear, then surprise, then relief (at keeping his underwear on), and then, oh my, good old-fashioned wonderment at how this previously thick, tubby young man turned into an Adonis.

Before he left that day, I added more words to my observations. I commented on the weight loss, the muscle tone, and even his erect posture. I considered throwing in a quick interpretation of the projective identification, but my thoughts were interrupted by Carlos, who said: "And, Alan, I wish you'd let me show you how to work on yourself. You name the time, and I'll meet you in the gym and teach you some of my exercises." I told him our time was up, avoiding acting out his invitation, per usual, to invite him into the superior, invulnerable position.

The *Critic* emerged early in the next session when we both had a chance to reflect on what had occurred. I said to him, "Can you see how you once again want to avoid being in the vulnerable position? You'd rather be the teacher than the student, the doctor than the patient."

Carlos initially resisted, reacting a bit defensively and saying, "Yep, I knew you'd say that, but I just want to take care of you, to make sure you stay healthy, to help you improve."

His reaction, here, contains a double dose of invulnerability. First, he will train me in the gym and, second, he will look after my health. In the ensuing weeks, we reviewed this episode and similar ones— each time subtly inviting him to let his defenses down and return to exploring the deep wounds he sought to hide. We discussed Carlos' unfortunate lack of an internal soothing capability, and how in the bodybuilding incident, he almost forced me to admire him. The inter- pretation led to a number of different growth-enhancing insights, as well as behavioral changes. Gradually, our work descended into the vulnerabilities he worked so arduously to hide. On several occasions, Carlos broke into tears as he shared more memories of abuse and neglect. He spoke, in greater detail, of the effect the family's many moves had on him. He was never able to make friends; he always felt like an outsider. He lamented the fact that significant others in his life, specifically his mother, father, brothers, and other immediate rel- atives, were not able to give him the admiration that he most needed in those early developmental years.

Most psychoanalytic processes, particularly involving more primi- tively organized patients, proceed with relatively frequent enactments of these types. So far, I have had four seasons with Carlos. Each one ends when he reaches his level of tolerance. Along the way, I have felt possessed by a variety of different, split-off parts of Carlos: the needy child, the abused child, the inadequate child, the abusive parent, the critical parent, the neglectful parent, and more. The episodes of split- ting and projective identification, inviting me into the *Exorcist* role, became less frequent. Carlos' ways of defending himself matured, and he also grew. Carlos has, over time, become more capable of discuss- ing his need and affect states rather than enacting them. Therefore, the possessions occur less frequently and, correspondingly, I now become *Exorcist* only on occasion.

Gilda

In earlier descriptions of her life, I provided examples of instances in which I assumed the role of *Exorcist* with Gilda. The most dramatic ones occurred during the post-assault period. During her fugue states, Gilda would first develop an intense state of anxiety, basically panic. Then, she would lose conscious awareness of her surroundings. She left her apartment—often at late hours of the night—walking aimlessly around the San Fernando Valley. She regained consciousness hours later, sometimes at 6 a.m., other times as late as 9 or 10 a.m. Gilda abruptly regained her orientation at the end of each episode, and then the panic feeling returned. It is little wonder fugue states occur in individuals subjected to extreme childhood or adult trauma; they serve the function of blotting out unbearable states of consciousness for periods of time. As readers can imagine, they are an extreme form of splitting. Once back in touch with reality, Gilda would realize she had left her daughter alone, unattended, barely at an age she could safely be without adult supervision.

I had strong emotional reactions to these episodes, the type of reactions associated with a concerned parent who realizes they have lost their child in a park, grocery store, or other public setting. I felt frightened. I felt guilty. I wondered if I had failed to see precursors and, as a result, failed to prevent these episodes. On one level, these feelings may be interpreted as simply the reality-based concerns of any treating psychoanalyst. On another level, these exemplify projective identification. Similar to Carlos, Gilda's mind became split. Whereas Carlos split off the part of his mind capable of admiring him and projected it into me (in the nearly-nude, bodybuilding scene), Gilda unconsciously disabled her consciousness. Her somnambulism blotted out her unbearable conscious pain. She was, in fact, amnestic for these periods. Even after she regained awareness, Gilda failed to remember what occurred while in the fugue states. In retrospect, I contained several parts of Gilda's unconscious drama, namely the frightened, abused child *and* the concerned, caring parent. I feared for her welfare—for rather obvious reasons—as well as for the welfare of her child.

As any competent psychoanalytic practitioner would do, I confronted Gilda with the riskiness of these behaviors once my own demonic-like fear reaction subsided. I told her I knew she did not consciously wish to harm her child or to create such intense discomfort in me. Additionally, and of course, I offered interpretations of how these episodes symbolized her victimhood at the hands of the assailants at her work. They also symbolized the way Gilda had felt in her early childhood experience, which consisted of frank abuse, sexual objectification, and neglect. These traumatic experiences created a fault-line in her consisting of barely contained emotional insecurity and feelings of personal incompetency. A typical interaction appeared as follows, with my leading the way:

"I can't help feeling, Gilda, that on some level you are trying to communicate to me the desperation of your own feeling states, especially their overwhelming nature." After she responded, or even appeared to understand, I would typically add:

"I feel some degree of your own terror when you have your episodes. Probably, I end up feeling some small amount of the terrific degree of pain, hurt, and impotence you must feel."

These excerpts demonstrate use of the *Critic* in conjunction with the *Exorcist*. As each demonic possession passed, I assumed the role of *Critic* through exploring the meaning of each episode. Some had triggers; others occurred without reason. We discussed the likely possibility I would need to file a child abuse report if the episodes persisted. I strived to present such a possibility in a non-shaming, non-judgmental way; however, I felt compelled to prepare her for the possibility. I explained the split in her internal world, validating the fugue states as primitive ways of coping with unimaginable distress. The role of *Lover*, always in the background, allowed Gilda to remain comfortable exploring thoughts and feelings she barely allowed even herself to know. These episodes also provided access to understanding what Kohut would call her poorly developed self-object function. Like Carlos, Gilda lacked much capability for self-soothing. Most people would find her emotional states, ranging from her years of victimization by her father's colleague to her being physically and emotionally injured by her attackers, unbearable.

I also took action between our six-days-per-week meetings. I contacted the treating psychopharmacologist, who, in turn, adjusted her tranquilizing medication. The medications, in conjunction with meeting her almost daily, led to the psychogenic fugue states emerging less frequently. Eventually, they stopped occurring entirely. Similar to Carlos, Gilda became more capable of verbalizing emotional states. She experienced many of these dark emotions in my presence. Often, they were accompanied by memories we would discuss in detail. These discussions bring to mind the idea, previously mentioned, that psychoanalytic consulting rooms function like time machines. Gilda would regress into the mental state of the sexually abused five-year-old, remembering scenes of molestation and reliving them. She re-experienced many similar feelings buried inside of her. She recalled the helpless terror as her father's partner entered her room at night and molested her. I repeatedly witnessed this, carefully absorbing her story of the sexual assault by the same man when she was in her early teenage years.

Slowly, over time, and with a combination of in-room work and the outside changes just described (like the medication adjustment and increased session frequency), Gilda became still more capable of verbally expressing these post-traumatic emotional states. Sometimes she trembled with fear and agitation while assuming these states; other times, she wept with abject sadness at the loss to which she had been subjected; on still other occasions, she expressed rage at me when I became possessed by the abusive parent, or the merciless assailants, in her perceptions of me. Through repeated processes of discussion, explanation, and tying in the feelings I had with the way she related to me and to others, Gilda gradually began reintegrating these feeling states into her own mind. Psychoanalytic work requires a great deal of pain tolerance. I feel immersed in dark emotions—fear, disorientation, sadness, loss, and more—even as I write at this moment.

In the months immediately after Gilda was assaulted, the role of *Exorcist* emerged most dramatically. The possessions grew in their power. By the time Gilda developed a seizure disorder, and her financial resources dwindled, I became possessed by unbearable feelings of helplessness. Arguably a result of my own fragmentation in reaction to her intense pain, I was drawn into the role of rescuing parent. Here, reiteration of my enactments, especially the time I handed her $400 for work she never performed, is limited by my own shame. Two of my "professional" behaviors—the brief employment followed by the payment—intensely validate the *Exorcist* metaphor. I literally became

Gilda's rescuer, perhaps even her savior, temporarily losing hold of my professional role. These were particularly dangerous possessions—for both Gilda and me. In a sense, I abused her myself by serving as the omnipotent parent (who could not, in reality, possibly be omnipotent). As noted, I eventually realized how much I lost my own way, got help for myself, and gradually returned our relationship to the typical type of psychoanalytic framing. Meanwhile, Gilda worked through her intense emotions around the failure of many caregivers in her life, including the ways I, too, failed her.

By the time we terminated our work together by mutual agreement, my assumption of the *Exorcist* role became rare. By then, Gilda infrequently used splitting and projective identification as defense mechanisms. Instead, she addressed the traumas to which she had been subjected, internalized the helpful parts of our relationship, and matured. She left depth psychotherapy a forever-altered person—the inevitable result of the serious psychic injuries she sustained. But the dissociative states resolved completely, her acute distress vanished, and her capacity for functioning greatly improved.

Penn

Various random factors affect psychological development, and Penn got lucky compared to Carlos and Gilda. He was born into a family that remained intact. Although he remembers his mother as "constantly enraged," Penn enjoyed a close relationship with his father until he entered adolescence. Then, he, too, rejected him. As noted, we considered this a "double abandonment." However, the attention Penn received from his father resulted in less early childhood trauma than either Carlos or Gilda sustained. Also, he enjoyed the good fortune granted by an excellent central nervous system and a superior level of intelligence. His parents sent him to good schools, and he learned quickly and well. These factors contributed to Penn's developing further, psychologically, compared to the other two patients. In fact, he displayed considerable maturity from the first time I met him.

It was because of such maturity that Penn relied less on primitive defense mechanisms like splitting and projective identification. Instead, he tended to use mature ones like anticipation, suppression, sublimation, and humor. Primitive projections onto me, therefore, occurred with less frequency. Although my role as *Exorcist* with Penn was less pronounced than with Carlos or Gilda, exorcisms nonetheless occurred. I assumed the role in several distinct ways. Perhaps most importantly, I identified with Penn, having been exposed to similar childhood trauma. I, too, had become rather achievement-oriented myself. Our similarities left me prone to pick up even subtle projections from him. Like me, Penn struggled to feel any sense of love from his accomplishments. One typical interaction goes like this:

"I can't believe the adulation I get, the awards, the certificates, the reputation, does nothing for the way I think of myself. It just doesn't sink in. I see it. And yet, I'm left feeling just as lonely as I have ever been."

Delivering the background attention and care of the *Lover*, I initially responded with empathy:

"I understand that about you. The external world of achievement seems to give you little in terms of feeling loved."

"Yes. I find it sad."

"I think it sad too."

Penn typically sat in silence after such exchanges. In the quiet, I tended to assume the role of *Exorcist* by enacting the maternal figure Penn never had. Partially because I identify with him, and also because of the intensity of the background fearfulness he experiences, I find myself in this maternal-like position most often. When not feeling like I want to take him home and rear him myself, I often offer Penn a fairly simple reflection of how he runs his life. I might say, referring to his repetitive, if futile, search for external validation, something like:

"Because you've done it your entire life, it's what you do. You have a hard time believing in love reaching you. You take refuge in being whom you think will attract it."

Often, Penn becomes tearful after I deliver such empathic statements. Difficult to classify as a method or technique, I nonetheless often just sit in silence with him as he ventures into the primitive, dark feelings of hurt and loneliness often emerging at these points.

A less common manifestation of my *Exorcist* role occurs on those occasions when I became possessed by Penn's internal critic, a schema we have come to understand together as the "internal Nazi." Sometimes, for example, I find myself feeling frustrated by the stubborn persistence of his over-achieving style. If I am fatigued, or in a lousy emotional place myself, I may unwittingly utter some critical words. For the most part, however, I can feel the criticism welling up in me and channel it into an interpretation of what is occurring between us. In essence, I risk assuming the role of the rejecting, critical parent—or at least I feel compelled to enact that role—an excellent example of the role of transference as well as of the *Exorcist*. The interactions often look something like this, and usually begin with Penn's own frustration.

"I was just asked to be the keynote speaker at the convention in DC, again, and I feel nothing from it."

My "inside voice" shouts out at moments like this, saying something like, "why the hell do you keep expecting it to matter to you, Penn?" Instead, and comporting with the idea that depth psychotherapists' work consists of channeling countertransference reactions into growth-promoting interactions, I keep my reactions to myself. I respond:

"I know that experience well from our talks, Penn, and I understand the frustration you feel at the endless nature of your pursuit."

Sometimes, anger emerges after I make remarks like this one. It seems to be helpful in that it vents Penn's internal frustration with his own repetitive and ineffective behavior. During these periods, we often have an exchange representing how mutative processes occur, gradually and over time. I might say something like:

"You seem angry now."

"I am. You should have been able to get me past this by now."

"You feel like I'm failing you."

"Well, aren't you?"

"I might be. Tell me some more about what's going on."

"Oh shit, Alan, you know the story. Nothing seems to make me feel cared for."

"You feel little care from me, either."

"You got it," he says angrily.

Notice the exorcism-in-process: By inviting me to repeat the compulsive pattern, by attempting to elicit my own annoyance (which, again, he sometimes does), Penn strives to release the internal tension, to convert the intrapsychic into the interpersonal. I resist. I let him stew in his own frustration, sometimes for minutes at a time. Later entering the realm of the *Critic*, I might offer a complex interpretation integrating information from the transference, his current relationships, and his childhood. Listen for how (on a good day, mind you), I bring together these three parts of his subjective experience. I might say to Penn, after I let the silence go on a bit, and the pain begins to envelop him, something like this:

"You've been repeating this pattern longer than you remember, responding to your belief your parents would notice you through performance, and continuing in your adult life, only to find yourself feeling as empty and alone as ever."

Depending on Penn's mental state, he might persist in baiting me into an angry, critical position, or he might fall into one of the dark, mourning states he must endure in order to grow past his childhood trauma. Here, Friedrich Hegel's[7] ideas regarding thesis, antithesis, and synthesis, formally introduced by Johanne Fichte,[8] become relevant. Only by experiencing these archaic emotional experiences, and being blocked from avoiding them through compulsive overwork, will Penn ever be able to ultimately relinquish the performance pattern. Meanwhile, I often feel tremendously sad for him. Sometimes I feel helpless and powerless, like I did with Gilda. Early on, I recommended Penn consult a psychiatrist to get at least some temporary relief from his extremely uncomfortable states. He obtained a prescription for a minor tranquilizer from his personal physician, and used the medication on occasion. Within a few years of our working together, Penn discontinued it. Instead, he took up meditation and aerobic exercise to deal with anxiety. Unlike my experiences with Gilda or Carlos, I never become completely possessed. When Carlos took his clothes off, for example, I wondered if I should have jumped up and told him to put his clothes back on. When Gilda had her dissociative episodes, I was filled with self-doubt as to whether I should have her psychiatrically hospitalized or otherwise intervene to prevent her from behaving in such a potentially disastrous fashion. None of these types of projections ever occurred in my work with Penn.

A final, subtle manifestation of my *Exorcist* role with Penn occurs during the times he becomes immersed in ancient, deeply painful emotions. It also qualifies as a type of projective identification because

I, too, become immersed in the same painful feeling states as him. The interaction typically takes the form of Penn becoming quiet, weeping silently, and then I feel similar to him. This is rendered all the more intense because I know these emotions well myself. Here, I digest his emotions—what Wilfred Bion calls the alpha elements—absorb them, and offer a combination of empathy and interpretations, allowing him to face these painful experiences and overcome them. A typical dialogue might look like this:

"I don't know that I can even stand this level of sadness," Penn might say, tearing up.

"I find it hard to imagine the level of pain," I respond.

Another long period of silence ensues. Penn weeps more.

"I imagine you felt this way much of your early childhood, feeling unseen and unknown. And the frantic rush to achieve and accomplish fails to bring you the love you so desperately wanted, and still want."

"Yes."

Years ago, Penn sought my help because he felt plagued by intermittent states of acute anxiety. However, over the course of our decades of intermittent meetings, we have discovered that the anxiety covers the types of despair into which he fell during this hypothetical session. Over time, the levels of chronic, as well as acute, anxiety have lessened.

After an encounter like the one I just described, I might wait longer periods of time to allow Penn to fully experience his underlying pain. Depending on the mood of the moment, I might continue with the quiet, offer more empathy, or even actively seek out memories that come to his mind. Herein lies the artistry of depth psychotherapy work. If I inquire too quickly, Penn misses the opportunity to find ways to deal with the pain on his own. If I linger too long in the silence, his distress might become unbearable. Every encounter is unique, regardless of whether it occurs in the first session or the 500th. Every time Penn regresses into one of his primitive states of emotion and memory, he works through yet another part of his significant childhood trauma. My blocking his access to his usual ways of coping with the pain—mostly ineffective ones he keeps repeating—a moment of healing, of transformation, occurs. The lasting change of psychodynamic psychotherapy may be understood as a culmination of these experiences.

Sometimes I share with Penn my personal experience with his types of discomfort. He finds this soothing. Over the course of many sessions, and particularly when he was in the throes of one of his "terror episodes," our discussions move into him recalling memories of his early childhood experience when he had felt precisely the same way. He often told the story of being the toddler of three or four years old, playing with a truck on the hard tile floor of his childhood home. He remembered his mother angrily rejecting him, cleaning dishes or otherwise straightening rooms of the house while he anxiously waited for his father to come home. These memories typically elicit great feelings of hopelessness and loss. Until we began our long journey together, Penn never imagined that any *other* could understand such extremely uncomfortable emotional states. I do, and each time we return to him reliving one, he grows just a bit more past their controlling him.

Reflections on the *Exorcist*

Various depth psychotherapy practitioners use different nomenclature to describe exorcisms. The pioneering theorists, like Freud, likely would have emphasized one-person psychology models, viewing practitioners as the vehicles for processing primitive emotions and cognitions in patients; the more recent, liberal theorists might view these exorcist-like phenomena as occurring in the field between their patients and them. I lean toward the latter viewpoint, although, obviously, I find the exorcism analogy helpful. However it might be discussed, psychoanalysts, regardless of their theoretical orientations, pay special attention to how the unconscious becomes mapped onto psychoanalytic relationships. These include how, through projective identification, patients project feelings states onto practitioners. They, in turn, utilize them as vehicles for transformation. Depth psychotherapists' journeys with their patients are nonlinear, dynamic, and unpredictable; the actual path followed depends upon each unique psychoanalytic dyad. The processes demonstrated in my work with Carlos, Gilda, and Penn comport well with Hoffman's concepts of spontaneity and ritual[9] in depth psychotherapy. My assumption of, and being invited into, the various states of possession represent the spontaneity of which Hoffman writes; the ritual concerns my relinquishing of the *Exorcist* roles and utilizing the *Critic* to subsequently confront, clarify feelings, or even use silence to enhance a resulting transformational experience. In the next chapter, I provide more details about how the *Exorcist* is followed by the critical analysis of the *Critic*—all while patients remain held emotionally through the role of *Lover.*

Notes

1. Foucault, M. (1988). *Madness and Civilization: A History of Insanity in the Age of Reason.* R. Howard (Trans.). New York, NY: Vintage Books.

2. Freud, S. (1923d). A seventeenth-century demonological neurosis. *The Standard Edition of the Complete Psychological Works of Sigmund Freud, Volume XIX (1923–1925): The Ego and the Id and Other Works.* London: Hogarth Press, pp. 67–106.

3. Stolorow, R.D. (2011). From mind to world, from drive to affectivity: a phenomenological-contextualist psychoanalytic perspective. *New Directions in Psychoanalytic Relational Psychoanalysis*, 5(1): 1–14.

4. Orange, D. (2011). *The Suffering Stranger: Hermeneutics for Everyday Clinical Practice.* New York, NY: Routledge, p. 30.

5. Klein, M. (1946). Notes on some schizoid mechanisms. *International Journal of Psychoanalysis*, 27: 99–110.

6. Bion, W.R. (1962). The psycho-analytic study of thinking. *International Journal of Psycho-Analysis*, 43: 306–310.

7. Hegel, G. (2009). *The Phenomenology of Spirit.* J.B. Baillie (Trans.). New York, NY: Digireads. (Original work published in 1807.)

8. Fichte, J.G., & Breazeale, D. (1993). *Fichte: Early Philosophical Writings.* Ithaca, NY: Cornell University Press.

9. Hoffman, I. (2001). *Ritual and Spontaneity in the Psychoanalytic Process: A Dialectical-Constructionist View.* New York, NY: The Analytic Press.

CHAPTER 8

The *Critic*

R eaders likely wish to identify *one* of these metaphors as most important. It would certainly simplify matters. However, the three roles support each other. They are entwined in a holistic, interpersonal process that uniquely elicits personal change. In combination, they create psychodynamic psychotherapy's transformative effect. The *Lover* provides the constant backdrop, the reception, and the sanctuary. Without a sense of caring and acceptance, patients would find the revelatory aspect of depth psychotherapy difficult. Some would find it impossible. The *Exorcist* consists, essentially, of psychoanalysts processing patients' projections. They *feel* their patients' internal dramas, process them in conjunction with their patients, and facilitate them editing and reintegrating updated versions. It is the exploration of such meanings that identifies the unique role of the *Critic*. Ideally, depth psychotherapists promote emotionally tinged self-understanding, effecting more transformation than achievable through only cognitive awareness.

If psychoanalysts-as-*Critics* utilized only verbalizations, the number of possible interventions would be surprisingly limited. Their quiver would contain arrows reducible to a few rhetorical devices—confrontation, empathy, clarification of feelings, silence, humor, or interpretation. Consider the idea of confrontation. One version consists of pointing out inconsistencies in patients' words and behaviors. A patient might sit forward apprehensively, appearing annoyed or irritated, but smile. A typical confrontation involves explaining the inconsistency, waiting for the patient's response, and facilitating more discussion from there. Practitioners may allow a period of silence to pass to emphasize a point or an experience. They might use teasing or joking about doing the same. Or, often, they will follow a confrontation with an explanation (essentially the same as an interpretation).

These verbal interventions are mostly self-evident. Empathy exists on the background level as presence (as in the role of *Lover*) but can also be focused. Patients reliving certain losses, say, of a parent or friend, usually benefit from their psychoanalysts providing a sustained, focalized empathy. Clarifying feelings, an intervention not oft-discussed, is just what it implies. Using this same grief example, the psychoanalyst might help delineate grieving from loss, or might even tease out some subtle anger at the departed person. Silence is one of the more artistic ways psychoanalysts work. Remaining with the same hypothetical, some patients benefit from their clinicians remaining silent when experiencing negative emotions. Others feel better hearing verbalizations. Herein lies another validation of the essential role creativity plays in facilitating psychoanalytic, transformational processes. Humor can tint all verbal interventions. It can lighten the mood or, in some instances, underline an important experience. I shall explain the final verbal intervention, interpretations, in greater detail soon.

Other methods operate concurrently on an unconscious level. For example, Bion introduced the concept of reverie,[1] referring to the way a psychoanalyst might have a "feeling" about an interaction, an intuition, or a seemingly irrelevant idea. They may get lost in a daydream, or even have dreams or nightmares, informing them of possible relevant themes. Many of these processes, unlike the verbal examples just given, do *not* occur on a conscious level. By way of an introduction, nonverbal possibilities are endless: Patients change seating positions, start gesticulating, suddenly becoming quiet or talkative, responding to an outdoor sound, changing their verbal prosody, and so on. These become part of the conjoint experience subject to scrutiny. In like manner, clinicians themselves could feel a muscle twitch, become distracted or sleepy, feel unexpectedly angry, or develop other reactions indicative of unconscious phenomena. I proceed to delineate some of the most common ways psychoanalysts intervene with patients before exploring interpretation, the most complicated verbal interaction, in greater depth.

Confrontation

Confrontation consists of challenging or questioning patients' presumptions regarding their thoughts, feelings, or behaviors. Existing as an analog to the immune system's protection of the human body, a variety of defense mechanisms keep unresolved conflict, unmet need states, unresolved trauma, intense emotional pain, and other painful experiences outside of conscious awareness. These strategies were identified by theorists as diverse as Anna Freud[2] and Wilhelm Reich.[3] Psychoanalysts commonly confront patients' use of denial, avoidance, suppression, acting out, and other ways of retreating or avoiding. When I introduced the metaphor of the *Exorcist*, I explained how patients with more primitive personality organizations rely primarily upon more archaic defense, like splitting and projective identification. These defensive styles prove difficult to manage. They often take the form of enactments (which, in turn, often require the *Exorcist* to untangle).

Confronting higher-level defenses, like denial, for example, is much like surgically cutting through skin to find the muscles and other tissues lying within. Confronting patients avoiding underlying pain through splitting or projective identification feels, in contrast, like maintaining a foothold during a strong earthquake. They elicit stronger emotional reactions in both parties. In any event, confrontations involve close attention and hard work. One of the primary ways the *Critic* intervenes is through the confrontation of defenses, which then leads, typically, to exploring what lies beneath them. Once the underlying issues are uncovered, patients typically need a more supportive response. Most depth psychotherapists acknowledge that emotion often emerges following confrontations. Such emotion requires empathy, the next topic of discussion.

Empathy

Lacanians, as a group, eschew empathy. They fear it invariably brings too much of the personhood of depth psychotherapists themselves, contaminating the process. They argue that, however much I might strive to mirror the sadness a patient feels, some part of myself is delivered with it. Most depth psychotherapists believe that, even if an empathic response is essentially communicating a cautious approxima-tion of patients' emotions, it still helps. They believe leaving patients in pain after confrontations is cruel. It is inarguable that clinicians cannot *entirely* capture their patients' feelings. They cannot help but include parts of their own emotional lives when delivering versions of empathy to their patients. Nonetheless, I respectfully disagree with these Lacanians, and consider empathy an intervention often worth delivering.

For example, a patient who frequently provides a detached, clinical history of his mother's death may become somber, even tearful, when confronted with his intellectual style of retreating. In the same vein, the patient confronted with an overly idealized, admiring impression of his or her romantic partner could, perhaps, discover envious or aggres-sive feelings underneath the overvaluation. As noted repeatedly, the role of *Lover* offers a constant background of empathy. Focalized empathy differs in terms of intensity and subject matter. Presence is constant, like background radiation; focalized empathy isolates the emotional state—whether it be anger, envy, or sadness. It represents another way of engaging patients, encouraging exploration or discussion. Sometimes, and particularly with clinicians with a relational orientation, they might respond with emotion itself, such as tearing up when a patient begins weeping.

The male patient who descends into sadness regarding his mother's death might, for example, respond to the tearful depth psychotherapist with associations to other memories. Alternatively, the clinician might, after offering focused empathy, request elaboration using questions like, "I'd like to hear more about how that felt to you" or "What was it like for you to lose your mother at eight, while still in your elementary school years?" Empathy might be delivered in other ways in the example of the idealization of a romantic partner. Here, follow-up questions could include: "I can't help but wonder if you have negative feelings toward her as well?" or "Could your admiration of her betray underlying feelings like envy or jealousy?" Assuming the patient responds in the affirmative, then empathy would, again, invite feelings to emerge in the context of an interpersonal discussion. Patients who would find such negative emotions disturbing may feel relieved by simply acknowledging them, validating that envy and jealousy commonly exist in the many-colored spectrum of human emotion and need not result in an additional layer of guilt or shame.

Psychoanalysts are often the butt of jokes emerging from the cliché-like ways they deliver empathy. They often use phrases like, "That sounds so sad for you" or "I have a hunch that felt devastating to you." Because depth psychotherapists have, for more than a century now, developed such routinized ways of responding, these jokes are deserved. Ideally, however, empathic responses are improvised to accommodate specific patient styles. Therefore, they rarely sound as insincere as therapists presented in contemporary films like *What About Bob* or episodes of *Seinfeld*.

Patients usually say *something* after psychoanalysts offer empathic responses. I once had a patient—another mental health professional, ironically—who repeatedly stated he *only* wanted me to listen. When I offered anything more than background presence or focalized empathy, he abruptly said, "Dr. Karbelnig, you're not hearing me. I'm not interested in what you're selling. I just want you to hear me." I struggled to accede to his limiting desires. I told him more would help him; he insisted my simply caring sufficed. Over time, I concluded I simply could not agree to his request. I wanted to offer more. He presented obviously conflictual situations, like a contentious relationship with his son. He resisted any interpretations, reiterating his wish that I *only* listen carefully to, and care about, the painful situation. I could not help but offer ideas which, over time, irritated him. He terminated psychoanalytic psychotherapy a few months later. Did I fail him? Perhaps. But the work always involves an intersection of two personalities, and I felt irresponsible limiting my responses to empathy only. Also, I feared I was enabling him to hide from himself.

Clarification of feelings

Most patients venture further than the ill-fated man who sought only love. And, yet, they still resist exploring their unconscious minds. I recently provided a year of psychoanalytic psychotherapy for a man struggling in his marriage because of his "extremely limited range of emotion." He could only identify one feeling state: frustration. He presented a variety of life situations over the year we met. I helped identify his reactions, using variations of confrontation and clarification of feelings. For example, I pointed out what I perceived as anger at times, and envy at others. I interpreted how fear of judgment from others (a projected form of superego) inhibited his experiencing more colors in the emotional spectrum. Repeatedly, I confronted him whenever using the word "frustration," asking him to consider other feelings lying beneath the surface. When he spontaneously expressed other ones, I assisted him in articulating them. By the end of our work, his range of emotional expression expanded. Unlike the last patient example, this gentleman completed our work with a sense of satisfaction and growth.

Silence

The *Critic* also involves knowing when to keep quiet, particularly when patients are feeling acute distress. Silence allows patients to experience emotions new to their conscious minds; it allows them to *experience* thoughts, behaviors, or memories associated with them. A patient who never previously felt the loss of her father, who died while she was a teenager, and breaks into tears after reporting memories of the loss, may be best served by silence. Even delivering a verbal form of empathy too quickly may violate her need for emotional immersion. Indeed, mourning processes can be facilitated by inaction. Similarly, it helps to allow patients to fully feel envy toward a friend, or fury toward a parent, or similar emotions. The simple experiencing of these emotions, in and of itself, facilitates transformation.

Lacan recommends liberal use of inaction to make "death present" in the consulting room, an intervention he calls "cadaverizing his [the psychoanalyst's] position."[4] He recommends depth psychoanalysts "introduce presence as such, and by the same token, hollow out absence as such."[5] Here, Lacan considers psychoanalysts as containers into which patient's project—an idea echoing Bion's work. Lacan believes patients' egos utter "empty speech,"[6] emphasizing depth psychotherapists focus on elucidating the desire of the *subject* rather than the *ego*. The *ego*, developed in reaction to parents' needs, exists on a distinctively different plane from the *subject*, which reflects authentic being. Psychoanalysts, Lacan recommends, listen carefully to patients' speech *patterns* rather than verbal *content*. Practitioners from other schools similarly attend to hints of subjectivity—whether tracking speech or silence, motion or stillness. One function of the *Critic*, then, consists of silence or absence.

Humor

Engaging in the psychoanalytic processes need not require patients to uniformly travel a dark, painful, tortuous road to transformation. Of course, the journey usually involves significant discomfort. However, the various forms of critique involved in psychoanalytic work, like interpreting dreams, repetitive psycho-behavioral patterns, lifestyle, aesthetics, symptoms, or any other conceivable manifestation of the unconscious, can be observed with humor. Sometimes, depth psycho-therapies desperately need comic relief. Carlos and I laughed uproari-ously, for example, after he completed his near strip-show and we had a chance to enjoy the enactment, in retrospect, together. A sarcastic comment may have a significantly transformative effect on patients. Consider a female patient with whom the depth psychotherapist has already established a well-worn pattern of choosing men who tend to neglect her. When such a patient describes being ignored by her current love interest, a sarcastic comment like, "Seems he's really into you like your other men," might well most effectively draw her attention to the problematic repetitive compulsion.

Interpretation and working through

Freud identified interpretation as the cornerstone of psychoanalysis. He considered it a primary way of bringing manifestations of the unconscious into conscious awareness. In fact, he adopted an almost adversarial view of it. He warned the "working through of the resistances may, in practice, turn out to be an arduous task for the subject of the analysis and a trial of patience for the analyst," adding how it is nonetheless "a part of the work which effects the greatest changes in the patient and which distinguishes analytic treatment from any kind of treatment by suggestion."[7] Interpretation remains crucial to depth psychotherapeutic processes as opposed to, for example, cognitive behavioral therapy (CBT). Psychoanalysts interpret the unconscious wherever it may appear, not only in the various ways noted previously, but in virtually any element of patients' lives.

Once brought into awareness by breaking through resistance, the transference and other manifestations of the unconscious become uncovered and are subject to exploration. Achieving only cognitive awareness of unconscious patterns harms patients more than helping them: They use their intellectual understanding to arm themselves. Practitioners' work with patients would last only a session or two if simple questions sufficed—"Can you see how you tend to pick abusive men because you were abused by your father as a child?" or "Perhaps you injure yourself as a way of drawing attention to yourself, which is unattainable through any other means?" Working through requires patients to immerse themselves in the typically painful affect associated with the unconscious theme, and experiencing new, reparative emotional experiences within the interpersonal context of the psychoanalytic relationship.

Michael Balint identifies the "two most important factors in psychoanalytic therapy" as "interpretations and object relationship."[8] In other words, psychoanalysts interpret patients' worlds—a form of critique—within the context of their work as *Lover*. He added the crucial interpersonal component to the interpretive one. A component of the unique self-psychological approach he introduced, Kohut recommends delivering interpretations *only* after demonstrating an empathic understanding of patients' subjectivities, writing:

> Every interpretation, and every reconstruction, consists of two phases: First, the analysand must realize that he has been understood; only then, as a second step, will the analyst demonstrate to the analysand the specifically dynamic and genetic factors that explain the psychological content he had first empathically grasped.[9]

The excerpt indirectly refers to the roles of *Lover* and *Exorcist*: Understanding comes from the *Lover*, and interpretations (or many of them) emanate from the *Exorcist*. The *Critic* weaves in and out of these two roles. Whether patients stubbornly resist, or openly yield, most ultimately become willing, even eager, to explore their private thoughts and feelings, to reflect on their behavioral patterns, and to delve into their unconscious minds—fully inviting the *Critic* into the consulting room. Lacan thinks psychoanalysts lend their desire to understand the unconscious to patients; however they communicate it to them, patients typically join in the endeavor, partnering with their depth psychotherapists in the discovery of self, other, and life in general. I explore the interventions described in the last section, in more detail, in two recent papers.[10]

Common themes in the interpretive process

Depth psychotherapy plays out in a dynamic, interactive, and spontaneous fashion. Neither psychoanalysts nor patients know in advance how sessions will unfold. Sessions begin like white water rafting: Psychoanalysts and patients approach the river with blindfolds on, jump into the raft, and ready themselves for whatever comes next. Perhaps they immediately enter a dangerously roiling stretch of the waterway; perhaps they enter an area of calm. Perhaps a session begins with one patient gesticulating wildly, speaking rapidly while expressing intense affect; perhaps the next patient, well into the process of mourning his or her deceased parent, enters the consulting room quietly and weeps in silence for half an hour. These ineffable factors make planning interpretations in advance impossible. Psychoanalytic practitioners play a role in navigating the journey but, as noted, sometimes lose their way. Naturally, they assume ultimate responsibility for the journey, however unpredictable.

Interpretation may be limited to the theoretical model favored by particular practitioners, i.e., Freudian, Jungian, or Kleinian. Other depth psychotherapists, like me, utilize a broad range of depth psychoanalytic theories in making interpretations.[11] They provide cognitive frameworks for unconscious phenomena (even though the interpretation, ideally, involves emotional *and* cognitive features). A conservative

Freudian, for example, might tell a highly self-critical person they suffer from an overly active superego; a Fairbairn disciple might describe the suffering as caused by a critical internal object; and Kleinians will likely utilize concepts such as "unconscious phantasy."[12] Those influenced by Jungian models may refer to archetypes when discussing the unconscious. Interpretations share a few other basic, arguably universal features, which I address, each in turn, acknowledging the incomplete nature of the list.

First, practitioners must be ready to react, to improvise, given the dynamism of depth psychotherapy processes. Ringstrom[13] believes psychoanalysts require skill in improvisation to engage effectively with the broad range of persons, styles, problems, and behaviors presented to them by patients. Second, timing is important, but also imperfect. For example, psychoanalysts might offer empathy about a particular emotional state, say, guilt, which the patient has not yet consciously accessed. The patient may reject it. An astute clinician will realize they should wait to explore that emotion further. Regarding the timing— another indicator of the reactive, artistic nature of depth psychotherapy work—Freud writes:

> Even in the later stages of analysis one must be careful not to give a patient the solution of a symptom or the translation of a wish until he is already so close to it that he has only one short step more to make in order to get hold of the explanation for himself.[14]

Freud here describes the subtleties, the nuances, of assessing when patients are near enough to self-realization that interpretations land well. We depth psychotherapists often have the experience of explaining an unconscious process to a patient once a week for a year, only to have them tell us they had the *same* realization over last weekend—exactly the same one we delivered fifty-two times! Patients are able to understand whatever self-destructive, self-denying, or even self-idealizing theme haunts them *only* when ready.

Third, interpretations carry greater weight if delivered within affectively tinged interpersonal environments. Melanie Klein,[15] working within a one-person model, advised psychoanalysts to pursue themes eliciting the greatest anxiety in patients. However, even this generality regarding emotional intensity cannot be applied as a default. For example, when working with patients on the autism spectrum, or simply those with highly cognitive personal styles, achieving a high level of affective contact may be difficult, rare, or even impossible. Worse, it might cause such patients to feel ashamed.

Fourth, the ideal interpretation, according to many psychoanalytic scholars, is one that includes transference (T), current (C), and past (P)—a TCP interpretation. Rarely will psychoanalysts tie together all three elements in a session. If psychoanalytic work is progressing well, such interpretations occur intermittently. Patients, and, arguably, their psychoanalysts, could not tolerate the emotional intensity of such interpretations every session. These experiences are powerful because they link what is occurring in the here and now (transference) with recent precipitants or triggers (current) as well as historical causes (past).

Fifth, although interpretations involving transference can bring depth psychotherapy alive, into-the-moment, some types of interpretation unfold within the spontaneous intersubjective dialogue developing between psychoanalysts and their patients. These typically emerge whenever the parties discuss the actual process between the co-participants. Psychoanalysts and their patients engage in intersubjective dialogue in myriad ways, including patients expressing love, lust, irritation, anger, or disappointment with their psychoanalysts. These often elicit delivery of more immediate, experience-near interpretations. Whether dynamically unfolding, eagerly pursued, affectively tinged, transference-related, intersubjective, or subtle, all forms of interpretation share one universal: They invite patients into an interpersonal dialogue, moving some of their intrapsychic world into the interpersonal or even intersubjective realm.

The psychoanalyst and the literary critic

In addition to the relational turn shaping how depth psychotherapy worked after the mid-twentieth century, a hermeneutical turn—referring to a focus on meaning, self-understanding, and even textual analysis—occurred around the same time. Orange refers to the "hermeneutic sensibility"[16] of psychoanalysis. She incorporated the work of

Hans-Georg Gadamer[17] in understanding the text of the human subject through the process of dialogue. Kenneth Burke, working during the mid-twentieth century and teaching such remarkable writers as Susan Sontag and George Steiner, offers insights into how literary criticism informs psychoanalytic work. Both professions concern themselves with the propensity of the human mind to create narration. Burke compares interpretive processes, which he considers "the fundamentals of psychoanalysis,"[18] as affecting patients by "providing a new perspective that dissolves the system of pieties lying at the roots of the patient's sorrows or bewilderments." He believes patients need a new, different vision, an "*impious* rationalization," which offers a "fresh terminology of motives to replace the patient's painful terminology of motives." Some of the interpretative process simply consists of reframing patients' narratives of their inner or outer lives. Burke continues:

> By approaching the altar of the patient's unhappiness with deliberate irreverence, by selecting a vocabulary that specifically violates the dictates of style and taboo, it changes the entire nature of his problem, rephrasing it in a form for which there is a solution. Insofar as it is curative, its effects seem due to the fact that it exorcises the painful influences of the vestigial religious orientation by appeal to the prestige of the newer scientific orientation.[19]

Here, Burke focuses specifically upon the depth psychotherapist as *Critic*. When Burke writes, for example, of dissolving pieties, he directly refers to features of the internal drama that are either disavowed, denied, or entirely unconscious. The new way of naming motives elucidates another editorial feature of depth psychotherapy processes. Whereas the above-noted patient example who has a negative self-image becomes accustomed to feeling bad about herself or himself, and finding others to criticize them, psychoanalysts deliberately disrupt these patterns by bringing them to the patients' attention. Also, and a definitive part of the working through process, depth psychotherapists facilitate transformation by declining invitations to enact these types of internal dramas in actual psychoanalytic relationship. They attack taboos by identifying the repetition compulsions patients cling to so severely; they confront and interpret the fear patients feel at the prospect of altering their familiar, painfully comfortable, repetitive themes. The change in the unconsciously preferred, repetitive style changes the patients' entire problem, to use Burke's phrase, and enables them to rephrase it and relive it.

The critical analysis of patients' unconscious dramas ultimately results in patients transforming theirs into one involving maturity and reciprocity. It facilitates the working through of problematic internal dramas, causing positive changes in them and, in parallel, in their external relationships, which also morph into more effective ones. Surprisingly, Burke refers to exorcisms in the final sentence, validating the role of the *Exorcist* described previously. Writing before the phrase relational turn came into common usage, Burke anticipated a more interactive form of psychoanalysis. He eschews the more archaic themes of abstinence and neutrality by suggesting depth psychotherapists explore, in a newly dynamic way, the "subject matter which has been surrounded with the pieties of intense personal devotion, awe and silence …"

In the final analysis then, we humans pass through life unconsciously creating stories of our lives along the way. Thus, and implied in previous chapters, an internal drama naturally has literary themes to it. Donald Meltzer, a contemporary Kleinian psychoanalyst, believes we either select people who comport with our internal dramas or we influence those who hap into our lives to behave in their assigned roles. If you consider individuals with particularly negative self-images, for example, they often tend to attract people who criticize, reject, or neglect them in some way, thereby confirming their internal drama. As Fairbairn correctly noted, this does not occur because we *like* or obtain *pleasure* from these internal dramas. We tend to repeat them— another way of understanding what Freud meant by the repetition compulsion—because we lived them during our early childhoods. They came to represent *home*, however uncomfortable. They are familiar even if they bring little or no enjoyment. Here, the interpretive process reigns supremely helpful. Keeping patients *pressed* against the absurdity of their maladaptive, habitual patterns creates change.

Having introduced the idea of the critical nature of psychoanalysts' work, provided details of the various rhetorical devices comprising their verbal ways of engaging patients, and extensively described the interpretive process central to the role of *Critic* and its relation to literary criticism, I now apply these concepts to the three case presentations, beginning with Carlos. I demonstrate dream interpretation—a key part of the work of the *Critic*—in the ensuing examples.

Carlos

Overlapping the *Exorcist* process, of course, came many times that I offered Carlos partial or full TCP interpretations. I described some previously, but provide a few more examples to flesh out the process. As I compose this chapter, Carlos has not consulted me for more than a year. However, he just called me, days ago, from a psychiatric hospital that admitted him due to acute suicidality. He called from the facility, seeking my assistance and leaving me this voicemail message:

"I just couldn't hack it; it upset me too much to see her [his prior psychoanalyst-now-friend] in a wheelchair. I kept thinking of dying. I checked myself in. Please come and get me out."

I tried to return his call within a few hours. Because of concern for patients' privacy, even "treating doctors" find it difficult to access psychiatrically hospitalized patients. Carlos and I then had several talks on the phone. A psychiatrist had placed him on a 72-hour hold. Only she could release him early. In my few telephone conversations with Carlos, he explained more about the situation leading to his hospitalization. Seeing his former psychotherapist confined to a wheelchair elicited thoughts of death and decay. His business success had waned, leaving him worried about his future. He moved to a suburb more distant from his young daughter but closer to his work. He distrusted his ex-wife's influence on her. These external life events culminated in him feeling unmanageable despair. Noticing him developing thoughts of suicide—highly unusual for him—he wisely sought shelter in a controlled environment.

The recent incident invites readers into another angle of Carlos' internal drama—the intensity of the core insecurity, most notably, and the many narcissistic defenses erected to protect it. Consider the meaning of these few precipitants: The encounter with his disabled former therapist reminded him of his own fallibility; even a temporary set-back in his professional success exposed the brittleness of the financial crutch he (falsely) believes protects him; his moving neighborhoods, while helpful for business reasons, deprived him of easy access from one of his primary projection fields—his child, his unconscious stand-in for himself. You might be ready for examples of how I interpreted these themes to him. And, usually, I would have done just that. However, events unfolded in a way which deprived me of even a chance to meet with Carlos—at least yet.

In our few phone calls, I reminded Carlos I was available for him to consult at any time. I confirmed he owed me no money. Carlos usually takes several months to catch up on payments to me between seasons; I have interpreted, and he agrees, how he uses the money owed to maintain a tie to me. I suggested he make an appointment with me. He preferred to wait, he said, until he was released. He asked if I would contact the treating psychiatrist in order to facilitate his more rapid exodus from the hospital. I consented, obtaining her phone number but reminding Carlos I would need an appointment time to assure her about continuity of care. He promised to call me back with an appointment time. On the last day of the hold, and in our third and last conversation, Carlos made a request:

"Before I make the appointment, Dr. K, I was hoping you'd pick me up here. I don't have a car, you know, and you're right near the place."

Taken aback by the request, and feeling perhaps manipulated, I demurred.

"I want to help you, Carlos, and I'm sure you know that by now. But picking you up at the hospital just isn't part of the work."

"It's less than a mile away," he protested.

"I know that, man, but you get my point. I'm happy to make a time to see you, even today, but I won't pick you up."

Carlos slammed down the phone. A few months later, he left me a message telling me he had moved "rather close" to my office. He planned to call for an appointment, soon, because of his growing concern for his prior therapist. I am still waiting to hear from him. I am certain that, at some point, I will. When Carlos finally returns, I will get an opportunity to interpret the interaction involving the hospitalization. It provides delicious examples of transference themes, as well as current and genetic ones. Carlos has long understood, as a result of our conversations, his propensity to project vulnerability outward. He will quickly understand my critique of the hospital incident, including the break-through vulnerability leading to the hospitalization, the exposed vulnerability during the 72-hour hold, the embrace he likely felt from it, and the triumphant request for me to pick him up like an Uber driver. What an amazing dance of unconscious themes! Carlos brilliantly transitions from such vulnerable themes as death, decay, and loss into reversals typical of the Kleinian triad of contempt, control, and triumph. He, alone, among his psychiatric patient peers, will have his psychoanalyst, a supervising and training analyst no less, interrupt his schedule, on the fly, to provide taxi service to and from a psychiatric facility! Ah, yes, truth is always stranger than fiction.

It matters little whether or not I get a chance to offer Carlos an interpretation of the incident. Many of his life themes follow the same dramatic pattern. I need only listen to him retrieve memories of his many awful childhood experiences that led him to adopt a "never again" attitude toward feeling vulnerable, and the opportunities for interpretations will abound. Because of his strange innocence, a guilelessness created by the infantile nature of his developmental delay, his behavior toward me—in any particular moment or over time—invites transference interpretation. Regarding the psychiatric hospital, even readers now understand the stimuli from his current life; the past has been repeatedly explored by Carlos and me, consisting of repeated abuse and abandonment; and, finally, the absurd request that I personally retrieve him—a complete enactment of role reversal. He wished to render *me*, not *him*, the servant and the slave. The situation makes a TCP interpretation almost too easy. He hands it to me. Carlos often does. Growth in him remains evident even in this example of literal regression: Carlos quickly exposed the darkness of his inner core of insecurity to me. The more it comes out in our sessions—along with the weeping, the tremulousness, and the shame—the more his deep inner wound heals. Like oxygen promotes wound healing, emotionally tinged discussion of psychological injuries lessens their intensity.

Unlike Gilda and Penn, who frequently bring dreams into sessions for discussion and analysis, Carlos denies dreaming. Of course, he dreams. His protestations represent yet another way he defends himself. I only remember one dream in my three seasons of work with him.

Carlos reported it just after we began season two. We had worked our way past his initial refusal to return, to the reparative phone call, and even past the "agreeing to disagree" on the issue of his insisting I promise to inform him of future medical emergencies. Carlos had just separated from his wife, meaning he faced some degree of distance from his daughter. Please remember his intense interest in Napoleon, noted much earlier, because the biography features significantly in this dream he reported:

> I found myself on a statuesque horse, proudly wearing my red-tipped hat. I was Napoleon. Hundreds of mounted troops filled the fields before me. I realized I was in Waterloo. My ultimate fate awaited me. I knew it was June of 1815, but the scene unfolded in the present. I realized Wellington's Seventh Coalition would defeat me. Next, I found myself in present-day Iraq, imprisoned in an Al Qaeda-controlled torture cell in which I could neither stand nor sit. An American traitor had set me up. He helped with the interrogation done through the cell bars. A Jihadist whipped me. The pain was unbearable. I was starved and dehydrated. I woke up to the sound of my own voice shouting, "Get me out!"

Here, too, luck allowed me the grace of a full TCP interpretation. Carlos and I were still freshly discussing the effect of my illness upon him. He remained insistent on reducing his session frequency to prevent him, in my view, from being too vulnerable. And, yet, Carlos remained freshly traumatized by my illness. His ways of coping with it seemed tenuous. I suggested the following themes to the dream: Carlos attained his perfect paradox of superiority and vulnerability in assuming the role of Napoleon in his dream. However, he also knew he was at Waterloo, the scene of Napoleon's final defeat. His fall from grace was imminent. The initial scene, then, represented triumph with a tinge of humility—not an inaccurate representation of Carlos at the time. I suggested the dramatic arc of the dream represents recent events, including the "traitor" likely being me and the prisoner standing for Carlos at the most vulnerable: trapped, tortured, deprived, and neglected. After enjoying one of the most effective and intense courses of depth psychotherapy in his entire life—that first two years of our work together—my illness abruptly terminated the momentum. It disrupted the process in a way reminding Carlos of his most archaic, infantile injury. He had trusted again. He opened himself up. Then, life shifted in a way reminiscent of how a betrayed prisoner in the Middle East might feel. In brief, the dream represents the transition from the shaky narcissistic defense, Napoleon grandly striding his horse, to the deep darkness of Carlos' personal vulnerability.

Gilda

Although also suffering from fairly primitive internal dramas, Gilda provides a remarkable counterpoint to Carlos' internal drama. Gilda's overt vulnerability dominated my interpretations of Gilda in my role as the *Critic*. The trend took its most extreme form in those frightening psychogenic fugue states, which solicited the most intense dread in me. When she emerged from these states, I typically intervened, initially, with empathy, caring, and, sometimes, silence. Gilda usually discussed her worry about the welfare of her daughter, and her fear of possibly hurting herself, when she presented for sessions after one of these epi- sodes. Often, after perhaps mirroring her first few words, I sat silently as her fear of what had happened in the fugue state slowly subsided. I only offered hypotheses of the meaning of these episodes when she seemed ready to receive them. I applied the cliché, relevant to the *Critic* in gen- eral and the making of interpretations in specific, of "striking while the iron is cold."

One of the first few episodes unfolded as follows. Gilda left her home, shortly after her sixteen-year-old daughter fell asleep, at perhaps 11:30 p.m. She wandered around the Reseda area of Los Angeles, meander- ing within a mile or so of her apartment. She had no recollection of the spell, and came to consciousness around 9:00 a.m. When describing the episode to me in a session later that day, I brought my careful attention to her experience. I let her reflect on the experience herself for a while. Keeping my own near-panic feeling in check, I then offered my empa- thy for how upset she felt about the episode. Much later, I shared my reaction of terror—another part of the function of the *Critic*. However, proper timing and artistry prevented me from discussing my personal reactions until the later manifestations of the fugue states.

Perhaps 15 minutes into any of the sessions following one of her "spells," I initiated discussion of what events might have triggered them.

I acted as a sort of detective. Gilda remembered how, shortly after her teenage daughter, Selene, had fallen asleep, she felt extremely alone in the world. She felt guilty at the ways she believed she let Selene down, delineating in her mind the financial losses, the illness-related absences, the diminished attention, the distraction, and other ways she had, in her view, "failed" her. Layered atop the guilt, Gilda felt ashamed of an entire range of her painful emotions. She felt shame at feeling guilty; she felt "stupid and histrionic" over her reaction to the assault, which was, in her view, an overreaction. Her thoughts turned to believing she had also responded "too dramatically" to her parents' neglect and even to the sexual abuse she suffered. Often her next memory, after sharing such an array of thoughts and feelings, was of regaining consciousness after a fugue state.

Usually, I would not have confronted patients involved in such acute self-attacks. However, we psychoanalysts risk aggravating shame— a type of self-attack, a feeling of inadequacy when compared to an internal standard—in patients already mentally assaulting themselves. However, because Gilda and I met five or even six times per week during this period of crisis, I felt confident in our interpersonal bond and in her capacity to receive ideas about the fugue episodes. In this one example, I chose to ignore the self-attack. I decided to let that element of her experience go unanswered, confident it would dissolve on its own as we explored a few hypotheses regarding what might stimulate the fugue state.

I reviewed the list Gilda delivered in this specific example: She felt isolated and alone as soon as Selene fell asleep. Next, she became immersed in guilt at how, she believed, she let her down. I pointed out the shame element of her reactions, including to the assault as well as to the more archaic injuries which shaped her personality. Dissociation may be viewed as a blunt, if effective, reaction to overwhelming discomfort. The resultant fugue state served as a means of, unconsciously, escaping her self-judgment. It also allowed reprieve from the extremely painful memories of the trauma she endured throughout her childhood, adolescence, and young adulthood. Dissociative episodes are most associated with severe childhood abuse or adult trauma of the severe, concentration camp variety. Completely overwhelmed by pain, the mind partially shuts off, isolating the painful thoughts and feelings.

Each time we worked through one of these frightening episodes, I would propose, only after carefully listening to her experience and allowing her some time to recover, that certain painful emotions had overwhelmed her, eliciting the vanishing episode. Often she verbally agreed or sometimes she nodded in consent. I witnessed her striving to integrate the information, to bring the pain into a sharper focus, to endure it, hoping to decrease the likelihood of additional dissociative episodes. I felt fairly confident in the accuracy of these ideas. An episode which occurred shortly after we began meeting nearly daily gave me pause. It happened on a Sunday night, causing me to wonder if the absence of the session with me might have had a causative effect. (At that point, we met every day but Sunday.) After a pause of some minutes, Gilda replied,

"Yes, I think so. I hate the idea of dependency, of any dependency, but I think I've grown to rely on you. Is it too much? Now that I reflect on it, I wonder if not seeing you that day left me more alone than usual, facing a chasm, a gap."

"You're the only one who can know that for sure," I replied. "But I, too, think it possible."

"I think so, too," she replied.

Here, I used the transference to bring the experience into the here and now. I succeeded, at least in part, because Gilda reflected on the dependency with me, faced the real-time discomfort of it, and, also, cognitively connected it with the other possible causative factors previously discussed. A person capable of great empathy herself—literally to a fault—Gilda clearly understood, consciously, my need to take Sundays off to rest and recuperate. My hypothesis concerned an unconscious dynamic. Because she received the interpretation so openly, I ventured one step further:

"I wonder if you might have even taken the day off as an assault on you."

"What do you mean?" she asked.

"Sometimes people experience an absence as more than an abandonment. They perceive it as an attack."

Here, I had borrowed a well-worn concept from Melanie Klein, who proposed a unique hypothesis about infants' subjective states. When left or abandoned, Klein believed, they perceive it as a persecution. They are unconsciously prone to feel persecuted even though no persecution intentionally or actually occurred.

"That aspect I don't see," Gilda replied.

I thought it accurate, despite her protestations, but pursued the idea no more. First, Gilda had already been rather open and receptive. Second, I took her denial as sincere. She was not being dishonest. And, of course, since it is her mind, not mine, she may *not* have felt persecuted. I remain devoted to the idea, even as I write about it now, because of the severity of the persecution she suffered during childhood, on more than one occasion, not to mention the assault, and now, perhaps, by me. Such cascading persecutory experiences could, in and of themselves, elicit the fugue states into which Gilda fell. Months later, after she and I had many opportunities to analyze them, I reintroduced the persecutory idea, and with success. She resisted, at first, primarily because of her propensity toward hyper-responsibility. And the possibility always exists that she agreed with the interpretation as a way of accommodating me. However, the fugue states dissipated shortly after Gilda could see how, in fact, acute feelings of persecution most often predated the start of a fugue state. Also, it turned out that more than half of these episodes occurred on Sunday nights. Surely it represents more than mere coincidence.

Several years later, as our relationship gradually entered the termination phase and I regained my footing in terms of the frame, I entered the role of the *Critic* in a particularly difficult and shaming way for me. I had already ended the unethical arrangement described previously and which my own guilt and shame can hardly bear repeating. As I helped her make sense of my acting out, and without justifying it in any way, our discussions often proceeded as follows:

"I wanted to explain to you what I think happened the day I lent you the money."

"If you have to, I guess, I'll listen to it," she replied with hesitance.

"I take full responsibility for losing the frame with you; that's all on me," I began. "However, I think a context exists that sheds some light on both of us."

"I'm listening," she replied, sounding irritable. "Go ahead."

"I imagine a cyclic process in which I like to rescue; that's on me. I can't help but wonder if, on your end though, there's a desire to be rescued, to have someone, me in this case, *prove* their caring to you. I think my need to rescue and your wish for the same combined. We ended up doing a certain dance together. Again, Gilda, it's my responsibility for it. It's 100 percent on me. Still, I think it a dynamic worthy of exploring."

"I hope you had a good time exploring it," she said, pushing me away, negating the idea while expressing her persistent anger.

"You're still angry at me for what I did. I remain so sorry about it."

"I get you're sorry," she replied.

Initial conversations like this one ended there, but later, they went on. Gilda needed time to vent her anger at me, to punish me for what had been, in truth, a significant personal and psychotherapeutic error. Nonetheless, in the coming weeks and months, we returned to repeatedly discussing the oscillating, sadomasochistic theme. Bolstered by Gilda's eventually coming on board with these ideas, and sometimes elaborating upon them herself, I later proposed that the entire dynamic might have reversed itself when she became so enraged with me. Of course, I deserved some of Gilda's ire. I *had* failed her. However, the ire turned to rage, and the rage persisted well beyond what seemed (to me, at least) proportionate to the regrettable departure. In essence, Gilda had assumed the role of persecutor, of sadist, in repeatedly lambasting me for my misbehavior. Sadomasochistic relationships often display such reversals. Quite often, the party playing the masochistic role switches sides, as it were, to even up the balance or perhaps to vent the anger of the slave, which typically builds up over time.

Not only did Gilda find these interpretations helpful, they gradually had a mutative effect on our relational pattern as well as her relationships with others. Over time, we tied in the sadomasochistic themes from her childhood as well as from the assault. Across those incidents, Gilda had been literally persecuted, violated, and injured. I pointed out, much to my own pain and guilt, how I had piled onto a process long-ago established. However, unlike any prior persecutor, I fully owned my part in the dramatic arc, apologized in an unmitigated and non-defensive way, and nudged the relationship back into one of mature reciprocity (mitigated to some extent, of course, by the power imbalance of our relationship).

Depth psychotherapy is far from an empirical enterprise. It proves impossible to weigh, measure, or in any way objectify what factor causes what, mostly because an infinite number of dynamic variables are in play. That being noted, I still believe, in retrospect, that the last year of my work with Gilda proved the most effective, primarily due to the complexities involved in the interpretations that emerged from my role of *Critic*. Our work illustrates how critical interpretations impact patients much more than solely cognitive understandings. Gilda passed through a range of emotional experiences during that final year: despair, hurt, neglect, anger, rage, righteous indignation, superiority, and more. She lived—not just felt or understood—real changes to her social role. Gilda transitioned from the victim receiving aid, literally and figuratively, to the angry prosecutor detailing my crimes and meting out punishments, which included threats of abandoning me (like she had been abandoned). Moreover, in the final months leading up to the termination, she had the *experience* of a mature, intersubjective, reciprocal relationship.

Most of her symptoms resolved by then, Gilda had found alternative work in a related field, and her relationships with her daughter and with men had remarkably improved. The psychoanalysis reached a natural end. She was well on the way to termination, as the term of art goes. You will notice how the change in our relationship had only persisted for six months or so—hardly sufficient time to create a presumably permanent change in personality pattern. Even with the reduced fee I offered her, Gilda could still not afford the sessions. And part of my recovery from my own lapse of judgment left me insistent that she pay me a reasonable fee. Gilda had incurred sufficient debt, mostly related to medical expenses combined with her loss of income that needed addressing first. A dream I had before one of our last sessions confirms the incomplete nature of the termination, and also exemplifies a countertransference dream:

> I am riding bicycles with Gilda for the day, well aware of the boundary-violating nature of the activity. It nonetheless seems natural. We are enjoying the scenery, talking to one another. After several hours, we arrive at an art gallery with which Gilda is somehow involved. She vanishes into the back room of the gallery. When I look for her, asking

the gallerists if they have seen her, they act surprised. They deny seeing anyone enter their area. Gilda had vanished into thin air. I react
with anger. I think to myself, "If only she would have learned to speak
her desire more, to insist on stopping at the art gallery or otherwise
making her needs known. I would not be stuck here in this awkward
situation, unable to find her."

The dream reveals my lingering guilt over the boundary violation but,
more importantly, my unconscious assessment of the status of the depth
psychotherapy. On the one hand, Gilda asserted herself and took off
on a path more authentic for her. On the other, she did so impulsively,
without discussing it with me (or any other), and without a clear sense
of the nature of her passion or interest. Only one potential interpretation, of course, but I take it as validation of some work left to be done
while, at the same time, confirming that much growth had occurred.
Terminations are always imperfect. I suspect Gilda will darken my door
again, but, for now, I reflect with delight on her growth, her freedom
from the type of despair she previously experienced, and the closer relationships she enjoys with family and friends.

Penn

My work as *Critic* to Penn helpfully contrasts with Carlos and Gilda.
He is the most mature; he was the least emotionally traumatized. He
offers the same array of dreams, thoughts, feelings, lifestyle patterns,
and personal habits subject to critical analysis as any other patient.
However, like most persons who have progressed well developmentally, and who generally function well, probing their unconscious
minds can prove more difficult. Together, we steadfastly pursue what
he called "the terrors" whenever he comes in for periods of psychoanalytic work. His underlying anxiety state will erupt, at times, into
episodes of acute anxiety bordering on panic. These are usually when
he returns. Penn has other problems, like the rest of us, but he can
be particularly resistant to depth psychotherapy work because of the
focused nature of his problem. When not feeling "in terror," he functions well and goes into denial about the underlying fault-line leaving
him always vulnerable to these episodes. He resists uncovering and

exploring other themes relevant to it, likely because his life patterns generally work well for him.

While Carlos suffers immense inner insecurity, which he covers with a grandiose shell, and Gilda shows a similar fault-line compensated for by excessive attention to others, Penn lacks a defensive style with obviously self-destructive features. Upon closer scrutiny, however, plenty of negativity exists. His is a slow burn of masochism, a gentler and milder version of Gilda's. He elevates one of Anna Freud's five mature ego defense mechanisms to its logical height, arguably abusing sublimation. Penn rarely plays. He always works. He feels anxious when not working. And, whatever pent-up sexuality, aggression, envy, or any other dark emotion becomes channeled into his preoccupation with achievement. He dies more slowly than the other two patients, but he dies nonetheless and at a quicker rate than he should.

One of the more common themes dominating my taking the role of *Critic* with Penn surrounds the old-fashioned Freudian oedipal complex—legitimately discredited by many. Call it what you may, but Penn often felt inadequate in comparison to his more successful father. He even felt consciously in competition with him. This particular internal drama is easy to spot. The Oedipus complex provides but one of many possible metaphors for the process of mature psychological development. Because of the frequent misunderstanding of the idea, I reiterate the key meanings of the stage. It describes the universal developmental process of transitioning away from the intense, two-person bonding experiences characteristic of infancy. The primary attachment ultimately loosens, unless destined to severe psychopathology, allowing children to experience intimacy with more than one person at a time. Ultimately, they develop enough self-sufficiency to venture out into life. Using Fairbairn's model, children pass through the bi-personal bonding of infantile dependency, enter a transition period (called the oedipal crisis by Freudians), finally flower into mature dependency. In this final developmental stage, persons remain dependent on others. However, they retain a degree of agency, forever balancing between what they can and cannot control in life. They know when to reach out for help, whether medical, legal, financial, interpersonal, or whatever.

The relevance of the Oedipus complex or of Fairbairn's transition period dramatically emerged in the transference during one of Penn's early periods of work with me. He came in for twice-weekly meetings at that point. His tardiness, which had been characteristic of his behavior during the one earlier period of work, recurred. He also returned to his tendency to begin sessions in silence or by saying, "I can't think of anything to say." I met with him for two 45-minute sessions at that point, and he often appeared 5 or 10 minutes late for each one. Most of those began with him sitting quietly, saying nothing. Initially, I simply pointed out these patterns to Penn, and reminded him of how they occurred, but less so, during the last period of our work. I told him I planned to keep an eye on it. I neither confronted nor interpreted his habitual lateness. Instead, by simply bookmarking it, I wanted to see how Penn reacted. He did nothing. He nodded, indicating he understood the observation, and then he continued to be 5 or 10 minutes late for each session.

Several months later, Penn mentioned, in passing, that he had learned from a psychiatrist colleague that my third scholarly paper had just been published. He reported it in a matter-of-fact way, adding,

"I suppose congratulations are due."

The compliment fell flat. I noticed the use of the word "suppose" as a modifier, and interpreted it as negative in tone.

"I'm not sure you really feel pleased with my accomplishment," I said, deliberately using the word "accomplishment" because he often used the word. Penn was, almost literally, addicted to it.

"Why would you say that, Alan?"

"Because of the modifier, 'suppose,' and what I heard as negativity in your tone," I said.

"I sounded that way?"

"Yep."

"I don't know why I wouldn't be more positive. I've published more than twenty, as you know, and I am regularly invited to speak at international conferences. I don't see why I'd be threatened in any way by your early success."

"Wow, Penn … you just said so much!"

"Really?"

"Listen to your words … First, you deny having any negativity, which, to me anyway, is pretty obvious. Second, you speak to your literally superior accomplishments in terms of work as a keynote speaker as well as having published more than me. I fear thou doth protest too much."

"Do I?"

"I think so, man. Notice also your use of the phrase, 'early success,' bringing to my mind the possibility that I could have more success, *later*, and which allows you to maintain your superiority over me."

"I don't need to be superior over you."

"I don't think you *consciously* do, yes, but neither of us can be sure of your unconscious.

Sometimes I think you feel you must overcome whomever you encounter, including me. It might be what drives you."

Penn paused for a long time, taking in the concept, feeling it, and finally said,

"Who can be sure? But it could be true."

At this, I felt satisfied that he simply received the idea, sat with it, and we could both watch, in future sessions, how it unfolded.

An entirely different level of work peppered our discussions, and a dream Penn once presented invites readers into what was also more of an experiential than a cognitive process. He reported this dream:

> I am driving hurriedly toward my clinic. As I draw closer, I realize no office exists. I switch routes, heading toward the home of one of my celebrity patients whom I treat for knee problems. As I enter her apartment, adorned like a New York penthouse, I realize several patients are waiting for me. I feel guilty at seeing her and the other patients in an apartment; I also feel anxious about not finding my office. I feel some relief at having a practice, though, even though it's at a strange location. As I begin examining my patient, she turns into several patients. I feel frightened. The group asks for help, appearing obviously in pain, and I begin weeping out of sympathy for them. Before I can intervene, they leave the office. I follow, only to realize they are following me. They ask me to only talk to them, not to do any procedures, and they offer a fee of $250 to do so. I agree, and they immediately coalesce back into one person. In the next scene, several psychiatrists from UCLA appear, tell me I am a skilled orthopedic surgeon, and acknowledge their familiarity with my celebrity patient. They tell her to let me work on her knees. She winces in pain,

and I again begin crying with her. She splits into three patients again, and they all seem touched by my pain. I learn that three other physicians operated on her and failed. I end up feeling frightened of them. The dream ends after I say I'll never treat them, and that they have hurt me.

After waiting a few minutes to see if he offers any spontaneous reflections on the dream, I ask Penn:

"What comes to your mind?"

"My terror, that's what comes to my mind, the background radiation of my terror."

"Please tell me more ... like what about the characters?"

Penn reflects quietly for a few more minutes, and then adds some details.

"The patient that turns into patients represents, I think, whatever audience I believe is constantly evaluating me. My loss of the office feels like my loneliness, my darkest fears—that the office I created as a mother-substitute vanishes forever. The psychiatrists seem like allies; they know the patient(s), and they know me. However, they recommend my proceeding when I cannot. I'm too overcome with their own pain."

"I see all of that," I said. Waiting still more time to let Penn ingest the emotion of the dream, I add a few of my observations.

"I am really touched by the pain you felt toward the patient. My guess is it represents the pain you feel toward yourself, the way you've suffered, the way you can never achieve a satisfactory level of admiration."

In response to these ideas, which I delivered with sadness for him, Penn fell into a deep state of loss and hurt. These episodes recur, intermittently, in my continuing work with Penn. In my view, each time the scene recurs in my office, a small level of transformation occurs. Penn becomes able to mourn for himself, for the guy-on-the-run, the man who can never accomplish enough. He sometimes weeps for an entire session, sometimes for two. During these periods of mourning, I typically say little and just bring my caring presence to Penn's emotionality.

One other common interpretation comes to mind because it fits well with the overall theme of my work as *Critic* with Penn: He uses his means of coping—seeking success, achievement, perfection—as a way of obtaining the love he never received as a child. However, as he has gradually become painfully aware, it never suffices. Penn often traverses the same repetitive path, only transiently experiencing feelings of accomplishment, and then he resumes his running, running, running. I have often compared Penn's life struggle to the Myth of Sisyphus, reminding him of his tireless pursuit of satisfaction through accomplishment. It will forever elude him, because peace will only come to him through self-love and acceptance of the love of others. These discussions can also, at times, lead to him facing the endlessness of the chase, its futile nature, and its inability to ever receive the primary love, as Michael Balint called it. My work as *Critic* with Penn consists primarily of bringing his awareness to his archaic, lifelong grief. As he becomes immersed in it, fully experiencing the pain of it, the inflammation around it lessens. He passes through it rather than around it. We work together in the shared hope and belief that such full-on encounters with his most primitive injury will lessen the pain—always worse in the imagination than in reality. Once diminished, the compulsive behaviors, which only temporarily salve the anxiety, should break apart.

The *Critic* forms one of the three key roles described, each existing in holistic relation with one another. The *Lover* creates the background inviting patients to feel safe enough to look inside, to surrender their defensive postures, and to enter into the transformative relationship with their depth psychotherapists. The *Exorcist* involves the transference, and invites the processing of all kinds of projections, soliciting more immediate, change-inducing interactions. And the *Critic* offers an overarching view of patients and their relationships with others and with their lives. In the course of this chapter, I described the primary features of the *Critic* ranging from confrontation, to clarifying feelings, to uncovering and supporting through empathy, and finally, and perhaps most importantly, through interpreting meaning.

Notes

1. Bion, W.R. (1963). *Elements of Psycho-Analysis*. London: Heinemann, p. 19.

2. Freud, A. (1992). *The Ego and the Mechanisms of Defense*. London: Karnac.

3. Reich, W. (1972). *Character Analysis*, M. Higgins & C.M. Raphael (Eds.) & V. Carfagno (Trans.). New York, NY: The Wilhelm Reich Infant Trust.

4. Lacan, J. (1991). *The Ego in Freud's Theory and in the Technique of Psychoanalysis. Book II.* J. Miller (Ed.) & S. Tomaselli (Trans.). New York, NY: Norton. (Original work published in 1978), p. 228–229.

5. Ibid., p. 228–229.

6. Lacan, J. (1998). In, *The Seminar of Jacques Lacan, Book XI: The Four Fundamental Concepts of Psychoanalysis*. J. Miller (Ed.) & A. Sheridan (Trans.). New York, NY: Norton. (Original work published in 1973), p. 46.

7. Freud, S. (1914). Remembering, repeating and working-through (further recommendations on the technique of psycho-analysis II). *The Standard Edition of the Complete Psychological Works of Sigmund Freud, Volume XII (1911–1913): The Case of Schreber, Papers on Technique and Other Works*. London: Hogarth Press, pp. 155–156.

8. Balint, M. (1979). *The Basic Fault: Therapeutic Aspects of Regression*. Evanston, IL: Northwestern University Press, p. 159.

9. Kohut, H. (1977). *The Restoration of the Self*. Madison, CT: International Universities Press, p. 88.

10. Karbelnig, A. (2018). Addressing psychoanalysis' post-tower of Babel linguistic challenge: a proposal for a cross-theoretical clinical nomenclature. *Contemporary Psychoanalysis*, 54(2): 322–350.

11. Karbelnig, A. (2022). Chasing infinity: why clinical psychoanalysis' future lies in pluralism. *International Journal of Psychoanalysis*, 103(1): 5–25.

12. Klein, M. (1946). Notes on some schizoid mechanisms. *International Journal of Psychoanalysis*, 27: 99–110, p. 107.

13. Ringstrom, P. (2010). "Yes Alan!" and a few more thoughts about improvisation: a discussion of Alan Kindler's chapter "spontaneity and improvisation in psychoanalysis." *Psychoanalytic Inquiry*, 30: 235–242; Ringstrom, P.A. (2012). A relational intersubjective approach to conjoint treatment. *International Journal of Psychoanalytic Self Psychology*, 7: 85–111. Doi: 10.1080/15551024.2011.606642; Ringstrom, P. (2014). *A Relational Psychoanalytic Approach to Couples Psychotherapy*. New York, NY: Routledge.

14. Freud, S. (1912). Recommendations to physicians practicing psycho-analysis. *The Standard Edition of the Complete Psychological Works of Sigmund Freud, Volume XII (1911–1913): The Case of Schreber, Papers on Technique and Other Works*. London: Hogarth Press, p. 140.

15. Klein, M. (1952). The origins of transference. *The International Journal of Psychoanalysis*, 33: 433–438.

16. Orange, D.M. (2010). *Thinking for Clinicians: Philosophical Resources for Contemporary Psychoanalysis and the Humanistic Psychotherapies*. New York, NY: Routledge, p. 14.

17. Gadamer, H.-G. (1980). *Philosophical Hermeneutics*. D. Linge (Trans.). Berkeley, CA: University of California Press.

18. Burke, K. (1965). *Performance and Change: An Anatomy of Purpose*. Third Edition. New York, NY: Bobbs-Merrill Company, p. 125.

19. Ibid., p. 125.

CHAPTER 9

Concluding unscientific postscript

S oren Kierkegaard, the lonely nineteenth-century Dutch philosopher, titled his critique of Hegelian philosophy, the *Concluding
Unscientific Postscript*. I borrow the phrase because of its relevance to bringing this exploration of psychoanalysis, and depth psychotherapy processes more generally, to a close. Kierkegaard used it
to condemn deterministic philosophies predating his own. A complex man, Kierkegaard was a theologian as well as a social critic. Most
scholars credit him with founding what later became existential philosophy. Much of Kierkegaard's work discussed what it means to live
as a "single individual." A devout Christian, Kierkegaard emphasized
personal choice and commitment throughout his extensive work. He
believed faith was an individual matter, a choice to believe (or not). He
proclaimed, "subjectivity is truth."[1] The phrase could equally describe
psychoanalysis. As noted before, any of the various forms of psychodynamic psychotherapy privilege subjectivity, not objectivity. Scientific
truth, or objectivity, concerns itself with propositions with no relation to knowers. Essentially, and to coin a phrase used by Nietzsche,
scientism deals with "disinterested observers." Subjective truth, in
contrast, consists of experiences obtained through self-reflection.

By definition, it requires the involvement of human subjects as knowers. Communicating subjectivity requires accessing one's inner self, and intersubjectivity requires the capacity to share such intimate, vulnerable, and private knowledge *with others.*

Working in their social roles as *Lovers, Exorcists,* and *Critics,* psychoanalysts facilitate understanding subjectivity and communicating it. Their work, too, privileges individuality, like Kierkegaard. As I complete the discussion of using these metaphors to understand how depth psychotherapists *really* work, I offer some philosophical reflections on the struggling[2] profession of psychoanalysis, examine the artistic foundations of the work, update readers on the fate of Carlos, Gilda, and Penn, and conclude with thoughts on psychoanalysis' future. But first, here comes a few words on why seeking your individuality, whether through depth psychotherapy, meditation, Yoga, or any other method, has become more necessary than ever.

The crucial importance of finding your individuality

As the journey winds up, the post-humanist era progresses ever more rapidly. Where is human individuality encouraged in contemporary culture? The negating, numbing, and erasing of the unique experience of the individual exponentially expands. The process accelerated while writing the book progressed, deteriorating still more so as it finally goes to press. For many years now, the cold steel of the audit culture characteristic of the accounting world has spread outward— like a dangerous malignancy—invading education, medicine, law, the media, and more. The importance of the individual steadily declines. Persons become symbols, numbers, and statistics. Learning, healing, or even justice is reduced to packets of abbreviated information or metrics of analytic indicators. Individual differences vanish, morphing into vast, impersonal, international trends.

Meanwhile, the media invades our lives like never before in human history. Even *The New York Times* and *The Washington Post* publish "sponsored content." For example, Mercedes-Benz recently posted an article in the *Post* about robotics. Only a close reading reveals its origin—written by a private firm, not by a journalist. The word "post-truth" was recently Oxford English Dictionary's "Word of the Year."

Educated persons no longer believe the veracity of information prof-
fered by major media corporations. They doubt the knowledge imparted
to them by their own educational institutions. Global corporations
track our telephones, access our computers, and inspect our credit
card statements, assessing our spending habits to present ads tailored
to our needs and interests. Such nonconsensual, constant surveillance
runs rampant, and space limitations prevent me from elaborating upon
what is happening in entire countries, like China, where such scrutiny
threatens basic human rights.

Even more horrifying, literal casualties result from these proliferat-
ing post-humanist trends. Campus violence has increased every year
since the 1990s, reflecting how technology, at least in part, desensitizes
people to the subjectivity of others. American citizens, regardless of
their histories of violence or mental disorder, purchase guns at alarming rates. Climate change wreaks havoc on weather systems throughout
the planet, killing and displacing thousands. The threat of nuclear war
grows by the minute. Tensions are the highest on the Korean peninsula
since the 1950s. Joseph Stalin's proclamation that a single death is
a tragedy, a million deaths a statistic, seems ever more relevant.

Depth psychotherapy hardly represents a panacea for these trends.
However, it remains the only professional service—and one with global
reach—devoted to the shimmering uniqueness of the experience of
being human. Even in remote parts of the world, depth psychotherapists
offer their services in institutes, clinics, or private practices. Those seeking relief from existential angst, diagnostically established mental disorders, or simply pursuing a greater understanding of self and other,
can consult a psychoanalyst. Unlike physicians, educators, clergymen,
or similar occupations, depth psychotherapists devote themselves *only*
to the agenda of their patients. The work results in self-discovery, which,
in turn, yields an equal degree of other-discovery. And, as illustrated
in my struggles with Carlos, Gilda, and Penn, self-discovery proves far
from easy. Inescapable forces, from early childhood learning experiences to societal effects, strive to change it. Even when we feel fairly in
touch with ourselves, or with others, our access to individuality can
be elusive. Novelist Amor Towles provides an insightful, poetic view of
individuality in his novel about personhood, *A Gentleman in Moscow*.
Responding to the question of what first impressions tell us, he writes,

Why, no more than a chord can tell us about Beethoven, or a brushstroke about Botticelli. By their very nature, human beings are so capricious, so complex, so delightfully contradictory, that they deserve not only our consideration, but our reconsideration—and our unwavering determination to withhold our opinion until we have engaged them in every possible setting at every possible hour.[3]

Ah, so true that, despite our immersion in the post-humanist era, the self cannot be reduced to a brushstroke. Paintings blossom in complex, contradictory, and capricious manners, involving media, color, size, impasto, framing, hanging, lighting, and more. Depth psychotherapy submits the self to consideration, and then repetitive reconsideration. Its practitioners unwaveringly encourage patients to reflect on their lives from every possible angle.

The dialectic as an overarching philosophy

In addition to the four philosophies foundational to depth psychotherapy introduced in Chapter 3, an over-arching organizational system—the dialectic—runs, like a vein in quartz, through them. The dialectic, attributed to Hegel,[4] and Fichte, originated in ancient Greek philosophy. Hegel's philosophy, much like trends in Western and Eastern philosophy centuries before him, emphasizes *process*. In effect, all things, including structures and functions of mind, are in motion. Three concepts underlie these integration-offering ideas:

First, as earlier philosophers as different as Heraclitus, Hegel, and Alfred North Whitehead propose, all things material or immaterial are in motion, unfolding, in process. Reality consists of verbs, not nouns. In fact, nouns are figments of our imagination, mere social and symbolic constructs. Jon Mills accurately asserts that Hegel, with his emphasis on process, brings "philosophical and logical rigor to psychoanalytic theory"[5] by rendering it dynamic. The mind, like any conceivable reality, is a constant flux of transposition and generation. Simply put, and as Heraclitus noted in ancient times, *everything flows*.

Second, although incorrectly attributed to Hegel (it really came from Fichte[6]), three words help organize such dynamism: thesis, antithesis, and synthesis: A trend or theme develops, another opposes it, and a third moves forward in the form of a synthesis. Hegel thought history moves forward in this dialectical manner. Third, and crucially, synthesis consists of a process of negating, in part, while at the same time maintaining what went before—a process Hegel called *sublation.* Sublation accounts for the fact, for example, that you maintain certain aspects of infancy, such as the capacity for terror or ecstasy, even though you are no longer a neonate.

The applications of thesis, antithesis, and synthesis are literally infinite. For example, the dialectic clarifies the history of psychoanalysis itself. Psychoanalysts have, from the start of the field, gathered into groups and schools, presenting theses at times, antitheses at others, and syntheses at still others. As I have covered in previous chapters, all depth psychotherapy models, whether Freudian or Jungian, self-psychological or relational, feature the unconscious and its manifestations in the transference, the repetition compulsion, and dreams. These constancies nonetheless morphed over time through the baroque music of the dialectic. The early one-person psychologies of Freud, Jung, and Klein focused primarily on the individual. Freud's dual-drive theory of motivation, and his tripartite model of the mind (ego, id, and superego) concerned the human person in isolation. Jung added the unique idea of universal archetypes emerging from the collective unconscious. He also proposed that a drive toward individuation, more than just sex and aggression, motivates us.

Depth psychotherapy models subsequently passed through multiple antitheses. The British object relations theorists, followed by Heinz Kohut's self-psychology (echoing Ronald Fairbairn's work), considered individuals in their social contexts. These theorists insisted humans are also motivated by social forces. Social fields pull them while, in effect, biological drives push them forward. Ongoing syntheses exist in the contemporary intersubjective and relational models of mind, and in contemporary models of motivation, such as found in Joseph Lichtenberg's variegated theory of motivation.[7] They offer more complex, multi-faceted, dynamic, and contextual understandings of the structure of the mind as well as of motivation.

As suggested by George Atwood and Robert Stolorow in *Structures of Subjectivity,*[8] each successive psychoanalyst after (and including)

Freud identified and named at least some unique features of human subjectivity—viewed through their unique lenses. They gradually created a fairly comprehensive understanding of the complex, dynamic features of thought, emotion, and behavior. Some theorists have coined the phrase "field theory" for their explorations of the interpersonal field as it transpires between depth psychotherapists and their patients. By implication, they also describe how it exists between humans in social environments. These represent further syntheses. As I explained in Chapter 4, Robert Galatzer-Levy[9] integrates concepts from quantum mechanics, relativity, and chaos theory to radically revise psychoanalytic theorizing. Reacting to limitations imposed by the static theories of mind characteristic of early psychoanalysis, Galatzer-Levy borrowed from contemporary science and mathematics, finding metaphors for describing mental and interpersonal phenomena. These, and similar models, incorporate some elements from prior models and negate others. The Hegel–Fichte concept of thesis, antithesis, and synthesis offers a way to understand the evolution of psychoanalysis.

The three-movement, dialectical concept equally provides a way of organizing psychological development. Each developmental stage involves a reaction to the prior one, an antithesis to a thesis, and proceeds to a synthesis. Infants begin in states of absolute dependency, but quickly (think terrible twos) rebel, crying out for greater independence. Ronald Fairbairn's concept of mature dependence represents a synthesis *par excellence*. The infantile dependency is negated, and a more diversified dependence is established. Sublation occurs because primitive dependency ends, while dependency itself remains.

The philosophical idea of the dialectic may also be applied to the quandary related to where to categorize the field of depth psychotherapy. Does it belong in the humanities or the sciences? Since the development of the scientific method, many scholars seek to reduce myriad disciplines into variations of sciences, thus, the evolution, for example, of the phrase, social sciences. In essence, though, such scientific reductionism requires a belief in naturalism, meaning the belief that all things in the universe, including your reading of this sentence right now, can be investigated through the natural sciences. Naturalism incorporates materialism, the belief that all things, physical or mental or cultural, are reducible to *objects*. In contrast, some groups within the humanities adhere to a belief system known as *idealism*. It holds that the ephemeral world of the mind, of ideas, of consciousness, will never be reducible to physical entities. Friedrich Nietzsche, like Baruch Spinoza before him, bridges the gap by considering mental phenomena just as real as the material world but irreducible to the purely physical. He proposes unification using perspectivism, as described in Chapter 3. In other words, while your brain certainly squirts neurochemicals as you read this, you are, nonetheless, having a real, subjective experience. Nietzsche, thereby, links the material and the immaterial, the subjective and the objective, attributing the difference to point of view. Along the same lines, Markus Gabriel, in his book *I Am Not a Brain*, critiques pure naturalism, noting that, obviously,

> there are necessary material conditions for the existence of many immaterial realities ... [But] ... the immaterial does not belong to another world. Rather, both the material and the immaterial can be parts of objects and processes such as Brexit, Mahler's symphonies, or my wish to finish this sentence while I am writing it.[10]

When viewed by clinicians and patients as co-participants, psychoanalysis operates in the world of the immaterial. Of course, neurological events occur during the structured dialogue, but depth psychotherapy does not *directly* concern these nervous system functions. Instead, it focuses on human experiences, privileging them as *real*, not just byproducts of the natural world. Such human experiences, like thinking of yourself reading this sentence right now, are part and parcel of the natural world. Gabriel warns that if we ignore the existence of mind, or culture, pretending that:

> naturalism in the form of futuristic science will solve all existential issues by showing that the mind is identical to the brain and that therefore nothing really immaterial exists, we will achieve the opposite of the process of enlightenment ... Modernity is ill-advised to define itself in terms of an all-encompassing science yet to come.[11]

Ill-advised, indeed. Psychoanalysis unites the sciences and the humanities. From one angle, scientific studies can be conducted on depth psychotherapy. Many such studies exist and more are being conducted. Jonathan Shedler recently conducted a meta-analysis of multiple studies of depth psychotherapy, establishing its efficacy.[12] On the other hand, science will never be able to reduce the immediate experience of a psychoanalytic interchange to an objective, scientific viewpoint. Too many variables are at play, from the individual psychology of the patient to the historical and sociocultural context in which he or she lives, not to mention the dynamic complexities of psychoanalytic practitioners with whom they interact. The *process* of depth psychotherapy resides more in the humanities, I believe, even though elements of it, such as degree of empathy or deliverance of interpretations, could be topics for scientific investigation. Regardless of its philosophical foundations, its evolution or its methodology, or even its residing in the sciences or the humanities, psychodynamic psychotherapy will remain, more than anything else, a form of art.

Depth psychotherapy as performance art

Depth psychotherapists' sense of timing, as well as their way of developing working models with their patients, requires creativity. They cannot apply theoretical models in a manualized way. Doing so risks confusing the map with the terrain. Human persons are remarkably unique, and clinicians' reactions to their individuality require spontaneity, reactivity, and artistry. More specifically, depth psychotherapists may be considered to be practicing a form of performance art[13] in at least three distinct ways. First, depth psychotherapists use their bodies in their work, paralleling actors' use of the cliché, "my body is my instrument." Lacan believes psychoanalysts give with their actual *beings*.[14] In addition to offering patients their words (through interpretations) and their desires (through the pursuit of unconscious themes), depth psychotherapists lend their bodies, their "psyche–somas,"[15] to their patients. They allow their patients to project onto them, using them as receptors, screens, containers, or, as I have discussed at length, *Exorcists*. Unsurprisingly, psychoanalysts often refer to, and write about, en-*act*-ments.

Second, much like the way painters feel apprehension at the blank canvas, psychoanalysts encounter sessions with fear of the unknown. Excessive anxiety early in an analytic process may represent possible, but not necessarily, projective identification of patients' anxiety. Usually, the anxiety has nothing to do with patients. Terrifyingly, depth psychotherapists encounter the infinite in every single session. As noted repeatedly, some patients speak of intense competition with their fathers, others present dream material, still others feel the envy and rage described so poignantly by Melanie Klein and her followers, and some experience hungry deficits of the type described by such theorists as Winnicott[16] and Kohut.[17] Any sense of certitude—particularly based on theoretical conceptions—risks objectifying patients. Psychoanalysts may be the *most* artistic in their openness to receiving, and spontaneously reacting to, the wide range of patient presentations.

Finally, psychoanalysts and their patients choose from an infinite number of possible ways of understanding the phenomena they explore together. Psychoanalysts' freedom to select from such a broad palette of theoretical metaphors provides additional support for the foundational artistic nature of their work. They help patients animate models of self that are varied, mobile, and capable of continuous revision, especially beyond the consulting room. Psychoanalyst–patient dyads discover widely divergent ways of viewing unconscious internal dramas, motivations, the meaning of compulsively repeated themes and of the transference. Most rely upon metaphors from the psychoanalytic opus, but not all.

I remember a patient who rejected a number of symbols I suggested for understanding his extreme deficits in attention. He vehemently, even angrily, rejected the idea of problematic executive functioning, an analogy I borrowed from neuropsychiatry. Unthinking, I took refuge in the horribly objectifying diagnostic term. The failure of my other analogies frustrated me. Instead, this patient told me he felt like the captain of a ship attacked by pirates. They assumed control over it. He viewed our work as a process of wresting control from the pirates. His metaphor guided our discussions for the next few years. He created it; he used it as a vehicle for self and other understanding. James Grotstein suggests depth psychotherapists "become immersed in the language of the patient."[18] What could be more spontaneous, intimate, and artistic, than developing a shared language with patients unique to each psychoanalytic relationship?

Artistry in the lives of Carlos, Gilda, and Penn

Human lives, as Nietzsche thought, consist of art forms themselves. Therefore, my work with Carlos, Gilda, and Penn constitutes art within art. Carlos, for example, required the most tolerance and patience of the three. He most needed attention and improvisation. I love working with Carlos. At times, his many criticisms of me, not to mention his repeated and sometimes abrupt terminations, elicited irritation, annoyance, and even anger in me. The artistry in working with Carlos involved tolerance for widely varied feeling states—in him and in me. I could not have brought exactly the same attitude to the other two patients; it would never have worked.

In our work together, Carlos offered some of the clearest examples of the role of *Exorcist*. Perhaps the most commonly described theme surrounded his propensity to elicit role reversals with me. In effect, Carlos frequently projected out the anxious, fearful, insecure "little boy" inside of him, inviting me to *feel* them. He succeeded admirably. At the times that I was doing my best work with him, I digested these projections and prepared, when the timing felt right, to reintroduce them to him. I strived to respond patiently and thoughtfully. Ultimately, Carlos was able to metabolize most of these projections, to take them back into him, and to mature. Innumerable examples of my work with Carlos as a *Critic* exist. Among the most prominent themes were the terrifically objectifying way he treated women and the fairly harsh way he related to his daughter (which will almost certainly bring trouble in the coming years). Carlos had a long history of projecting an idealized version of himself onto his daughter, having extremely high expectations for her academic performance and even moral behavior.

Gilda ultimately required great patience from me as well, but only after the assault. She needed close, intimate caring, and fairly aggressive interpretations initially. The extremely difficult combination of severe childhood trauma, whatever neurobiological vulnerabilities existed, and exposure to a severe assault during adulthood, proved a great challenge to our work together. Improvisation was needed along the way, essentially on a session-by-session basis. Adhering to the basic frame of the loving, holding environment, to use Winnicott's phrase, proved not only difficult but dangerous. Gilda and I shared many common interests in the realms of literature, philosophy, history, and music. I had to exert great self-control to keep my physical attraction to her in check—another artistic skill. Knowing the extremely self-destructive nature of any sexual enactments, my struggle lessened over time. However, and as painfully described in several earlier parts of this book, it peaked in the months after she was attacked. Also, as the psychogenic fugues persisted, arousing terrific fear in both of us, my concern for her well-being ultimately overshadowed my erotic attraction to her.

The fugue states provide a transition to understanding the ways I served as an *Exorcist* for Gilda. In her most regressed moments, I became the agent for her near-totally absent ego. Gilda literally lost her conscious experience for hours at a time, wandering around the Reseda area and placing her personal safety at risk. I actively intervened, considering psychiatric hospitalization and discussing her status with the treating psychiatrist. Fortunately, the psychiatrist and I, together, were able to contain Gilda's distress without resorting to a psychiatric hospitalization. Another example of exorcism exists within my physical attraction itself. I harbor an intense wish to rescue others. A seemingly perfect match for such a trend, Gilda projects a helpless, needy self in need of protection. I also took possession of this part of her. Fortunately for both of us, I was—eventually—able to absorb and translate these experiences, namely my desire to rescue in combination with her need for such rescue, into our discussions. These highly nuanced experiences also characterize the artistry of psychoanalytic work. No manual could ever describe how to react to such unusual psychological phenomena as unfolded between Gilda and me.

My work as the *Critic* of Gilda's life ranged far and wide. It included the way that she parented her daughter, how she managed her lawsuit related to the physical assault against her employer, and her relationship with many others—potential suitors, friends, family, administrative officials, attorneys, and treating physicians. We devoted a great deal of time to her romantic relationships, particularly because they had such remarkable sadomasochistic themes. The *Critic* requires artistry mostly in terms of timing. However, experience also provides knowledge of common self-destructive trends in human beings, much like experience with painting imbues artists with knowledge of color theory. With Gilda, I faced the dangerous combination of my own personal vulnerabilities, my deep romantic attraction to her, and her extremely severe psychological disturbances. I have a part-time forensic practice as well as one focusing on depth psychotherapy. As a result, I have considerable experience with boundary violations by clinical practitioners of all stripes. The types of boundary crossing I described often occur, as do overt sexual enactments. I learned from my work with Gilda that no one is immune from such enactments. It was humbling, and reviewing the experience through writing about her brought up residuals of shame with which I shall struggle for the rest of my life.

I, too, experienced separation anxiety when I first went off to college. Although the anxiety I experienced did not approach the level of the panic attacks Penn described, I certainly identified with many of his life struggles. This identification process facilitated my creating a warm, embracing environment for him. Because of the less primitive nature of Penn's psychological organization, I did not have to fight off the competition I felt, at times, with Carlos or the profound urge to rescue I felt with Gilda. Also, because of his maturity, the possibilities for exorcism were less dramatic in Penn's case. They nonetheless occurred. Most commonly, I felt the anxiety of which Penn complained, a combination of his process and mine. I received the projection of his hopelessness—much like possession by a devil—processing it, interpreting it, and extensively discussing it with him. Penn became more hopeful when he could see, slowly, gradually, almost glacially, positive changes occurring. Over time, the projections diminished. I also received his projection of the omnipotent caregiver, the one *finally* capable of seeing the awesomeness of his many accomplishments. Although I admired him, and validated his successes, I also behaved like an *Exorcist* by receiving that specific projection. We worked through it, over months and years, until he learned, and grieved, how his compulsive adherence to achievement would never provide him with the love he never received. Instead of being so driven to accomplish, Penn needed to face the loss, to weep and moan and shriek. Regarding the psychoanalyst as *Critic*, Penn and I focused primarily on a variety of the old-fashioned concept of the Oedipus complex. Penn struggled mightily to create an identity that was just as good as, but strikingly different from, his father's. I once asked him if he could imagine being buried in a different place than alongside his father—an intervention intended to dramatically get his attention. He burst into tears.

The chronic incompleteness of depth psychotherapy work

None of the three patients I presented ended their work with me in ideal ways. Carlos has changed for the positive in many, even potentially measurable ways. He completely relinquished his excessive reliance upon drugs and alcohol. He integrated his previously impulsive ways of being in the world with a more mature, deliberative one, allowing him to resolve problems with the IRS and to become more efficient and successful. However, he continues to struggle with trusting others. He lacks any real friendships. As evident in his application of the word "seasons" to our various periods of work together, he can only bear so much exposure to his wounded inner core. If he were to never consult me or any other depth psychotherapist, conclusions reached regarding his progress, or even his overall maturity, would be mixed. Carlos has certainly felt satisfied with our meetings, and often reminds me during our off times of his intention to return. He has not yet returned, but I expect he will.

Much like Carlos, Gilda, too, made significant gains. They seem to be more significant and longer lasting than his. She recovered considerably from the early childhood and more recent trauma, although scarring will inevitably remain. Her masochistic style underwent a shift in severity. While still prone to devaluing herself and sacrificing excessively, her relationship with her daughter, with her friends, with men, and with her coworkers and supervisors has generally matured. Like Carlos, she, too, feels satisfied with the work. As she rebuilds her financial life, she may return for more depth psychotherapeutic work. However, I would not be surprised if my role in further traumatizing her—however briefly— may be unforgivable to her. I have yet to fully forgive myself. I would not blame her if she chooses never to meet with me again. And, in any event, the termination of our work resulted more from financial than from "full closure" reasons.

Penn has made the most positive progress of the three patients, but he, too, remains in flux. Like Carlos, he plans on consulting me intermittently, "until death do us part," as he often says. I, or we, cannot fully take responsibility for his positive gains. Penn began intermittent depth psychotherapy nearly thirty-five years ago after enjoying a basically stable childhood environment and inheriting basically sound neuropsychiatric functioning. Whereas both Carlos and Gilda could be considered examples of persons with personality disorders (narcissistic and borderline, respectively), Penn has no such foundational disorder. Our work over the course of many years reminds me of Michael Balint's simple binary of the healing centrality of the professional relationship and interpretations. Penn has benefited from a type of re-parenting, an internalization of the relationship with me that has clearly lessened the deficit in his ability for self-soothing. His anxiety spells occur with less frequency and intensity. He has an extensive cognitive understanding of the ways he was traumatized, and perhaps most significantly, of how his ardent devotion to work and productivity only temporarily salves his mental pain. In addition to feeling less anxiety, Penn has become, over time, less reliant on those coping patterns. He has developed some distinct, non-work-related interests, like bird watching and exercising. His capacity for intimacy is greatly improved, as demonstrated in the closeness he enjoys with his wife and his two sons.

Reflecting on my nearly four decades of clinical experience, the way depth psychotherapies typically end invites humility. I estimate only one-third of patients terminate in a full, comprehensive way in which specific goals are accomplished, both parties have time to review these changes, and the work comes to a mutually agreed-upon ending. None of the three persons whose lives I present here ended their work with me in this ideal fashion. Many patients have, but not these three. Even this conclusion is subject to alteration depending on one's perspective, though. In many senses, each ending with Carlos and Penn constituted a full termination, with goals achieved at the time and even a shared understanding of what changes would be desirable in the future.

Another third of patients end depth psychotherapy in the way Gilda did. A natural end-point emerges. With her, it occurred after I re-established proper boundaries with her and further gains were achieved. A few years later, it became evident to both of us that she simply could not afford to continue financially. We had plenty of time to discuss the termination. We shared similar viewpoints about goals achieved, changes made, and lifestyles altered. And, yet, even that ending was far from ideal. She remained angry at me until the very last session. We both felt additional work would help her to consolidate the gains she made and to push her toward greater self-acceptance and a greater capacity for self-actualization.

The other third of patients end in ways all parties would agree are incomplete. These occur for a variety of reasons. Sometimes financial resources are exhausted before desired results are achieved. Sometimes patients become angry, dissatisfied, annoyed, and incapable of working through their negative feelings. Sometimes depth psychotherapists make unforgivable mistakes, caring too much, for example, or too little, or engaging in destructive boundary violations. Often, patients run into a thought-process, or an emotional state, simply too unbearable for them to endure. If Carlos did not remain so involved in our work, for example, any of the endings of our seasons of work would fit into just such a negative category. The seasons have typically ended because of the reason noted: Carlos becomes too upset by confronting the depth of his own despair. He cannot bear feeling it; he loses his desire to explore it. Other patients end depth psychotherapy work for similar reasons, or because they encounter homosexual longings, homicidal urges, panic feelings, or other intensely uncomfortable psycho-physiological states that they feel are better served by avoiding further introspection. But, then again, is it possible that even so-called objective indicators, like destroying bacterial infections, are ultimately temporary anyway?

A warning to depth psychotherapy practitioners and patients

Should you contemplate consulting a depth psychotherapist, proceed with caution. Although we depth psychotherapists deliver informed consent forms like our medical and legal colleagues, the potential side-effects of the work, if fully delineated, would fill volumes. Injured persons entering depth psychotherapists' offices will almost certainly exit, perhaps without acute despair and inflammation, but still-injured. The abuse by their childhood neighbor, the attack by muggers, the loss of a child to cancer—those facts of life never go away. Trauma cannot be undone. Patients only partially recover from these wounds. They learn to go on living. And those with personality disorders may reduce their intensity, but they will continue to veer toward whatever the extremity may be, whether narcissism, masochism, dependency, or wherever. People change. But, perhaps their attitude toward themselves changes the most. In any event, and however patients morph, their growth typically betrays efforts to evaluate it. How can you measure subtle increases in self-valuation, in sensitivity to others, in resistance to abusive relationships? No red blood cell test, effectively determining a level of anemia, exists for the mind. We are, as Towles noted, too capricious, too complex.

The same types of complications, in reverse, affect practitioners of psychoanalysis. Like the patients who consult them, depth psychotherapists view their patients through their own unique perspectives, influenced by their historical, sociocultural, personal, and other individualistic factors. They strive to maintain an even-handed focus on information emanating from patients, but must, of necessity, view them through their own lenses and biases. On the one hand, depth psychotherapists' powers are immense: They facilitate an encounter with human subjectivity unequaled by any other profession. They break through defenses, exposing patients to any number of conflicts, memories, and traumas of which they were previously unaware. Along the way, they dig through painful emotional states, love and loss, rage and despair, unsatisfied longings, unresolved heartbreaks, nameless dread, and endless others. As a result of the realizations, particularly the interpersonal patterns discovered in the transference and other relationships, patients often make relational changes. They may grow closer to their spouses; they may divorce them. They may end friendships; they start others. They may become more invested in their occupations, or they may transition into another one.

On the other hand, depth psychotherapists, unlike their medical colleagues, lack any true power. Unlike the surgeon, they cannot remove cancerous tissues. Unlike the anesthetist, they cannot directly eliminate pain. They work within the dialectic of power and helplessness, offering patients information within the context of a transformative relationship. Patients remain agents of their lives. If anything, depth psychotherapy works to increase their personal agency and authority, but it is ultimately up to *them*, not their psychoanalysts, to make whatever changes they wish in their lives. I often tell patients, when orienting them to the depth psychotherapy process, that the only direct advice

I will give them is to avoid jumping off a bridge. The rest of their life decisions are up to them.

These reflections lead me to comment on the qualities required for working as practitioners of depth psychotherapy. Clinicians need a deep capacity for empathy. They require an openness to the many varied ways human persons experience their lives. Ideally, they find humans interesting. They feel intrigued by the variations in how patients love, work, and play. They are interested in human psychology, in the world of the mind. Depth psychotherapists must, on the one hand, acquaint themselves with the power of transformation while, on the other hand, be ready to have little or no impact on people. Perhaps the paradox of power and powerlessness is the most humbling aspect of the work.

The future of depth psychotherapy

Where does depth psychotherapy go from here, given the global regression to scientism and empiricism? Time will tell. The violence, alienation, and isolation endemic to the contemporary world will probably lead more people to consult psychoanalytic clinicians to help them learn more about themselves, to facilitate their emergent individuality, and to celebrate their clarity in visions of self, other, and the world. Record levels of mental health disturbances already plague the planet. The most recent version of the *Diagnostic and Statistical Manual*, published by the American Psychiatric Association, estimates some 25 percent of Americans will suffer from a diagnosable mental disorder at some point in their lives. Meanwhile, in those lacking formal diagnoses, cultural forces like technology, social media, media manipulation, income inequality, and global warming have already, and will continue to, create unprecedented feelings of alienation. People will feel increasingly alone, misunderstood, and unloved. They will yearn for self-exploration to free themselves from the tyranny of the many trends ever separating their subject, as Lacan would call it, from their ego. Their egos are increasingly poisoned.

Meanwhile, the drive for self-knowledge persists, as usual. Carl Linnaeus, the biologist who named our species *Homo sapiens*, considered human beings' characteristic feature the desire for self-knowledge. He cites Socrates' admonition to "know thyself!"[19] For Linnaeus, then, what makes us human is precisely our status as *sapiens*, as living beings capable of wisdom. Between the cultural forces eliciting alienation, and such elements of our essential human nature, psychoanalysts will never lack patients. Given the sociocultural forces just noted, they will, instead, likely cascade into their offices.

A more serious problem exists in the organization of the depth psychotherapy project itself. From the onset, it has been plagued by infighting. Even today, no cohesive model for psychoanalysis exists. According to Steven Pinker, the Harvard-based evolutionary psychologist, we humans will forever be prone to forming us-versus-them dichotomies, and, thus, the history of Jung splitting from Freud, Fairbairn from Klein, and on and on endlessly. The many psychoanalytic schools and groups claiming supremacy scattered around the globe will likely continue forever. The unfortunate fragmentation in depth psychotherapy theories seems endemic.

However, after more than a century of existence, trends toward unification and cohesion are beginning to appear. Consistent with Hegel's and Fiche's idea that history moves forward through a dialectical process, psychoanalysts such as Leo Rangell,[20] Wallerstein, Jay, Stepansky,[21] and Arnold Goldberg,[22] call for more of an emphasis on commonalities, as I have. A new synthesis is emerging. Of course, other theorists will quibble with my nomenclature, and offer alternative terms, but none can disagree with the premise that, whatever you call it, and regardless of the metaphors they use, depth psychotherapists *frame* their relationships with patients, bring their emotional *presence* to them, and *engage* with them in a variety of ways, all intending to foment personal transformation.

Depth psychotherapists need not consist of angry groups sporting unfounded and unnecessary antipathies toward one another. Ideally, the field will remain a highly personal, individualized way of helping people suffer less pain and enjoy more freedom, and its practitioners will acknowledge similarities, like in how they all use a similar method regardless of theoretical preference. Depth psychotherapies allegedly reducible to a three-letter acronyms (TLA), like Emotionally Focused Therapy (EFT), Transference Focused Therapy (TFT), or the longer-termed Intensive Short-Term Dynamic Psychotherapy (ISTDP), should be steadfastly avoided. Although the practitioners of these methods are well-intended, and often well-trained, they risk becoming trapped in the ideology of their methods. In focusing any therapy on the emotions, for example, depth psychotherapists may violate patients by holding emotional expectations for them. Each psychoanalytic session is unique. Psychoanalytic performances can be neither duplicated nor mechanized. They cannot be reduced to algorithmic manuals. I have repeatedly noted that, of course, clinicians cannot be entirely freed from bias. But they ideally have received substantial depth psychotherapy themselves. They have a sense of their own predispositions and, in any event, avoid adopting any methodology which restrains patients. They must remain permanently humbled by the complexity of human subjectivity, and by the degree of ignorance that *always* remains about themselves and others.

Concluding finally with a sample of how an initial depth psychotherapy encounter might unfold, imagine you enter the well-furnished, quiet room of a practitioner, ready to reduce your sadness, address your conflict-laden relationship, or explore your dreams. You start unsure of how to proceed, and ask the clinician:

"How should I begin?"

"It's up to you," the psychoanalyst might say. "No specific agenda exists."

A pause ensues. The practitioner faces a choice point—allow more silence or intervene with some questions? In this case, she senses discomfort in the patient and chooses to draw him or her out.

"What's on your mind?"

And so the adventure begins.

Notes

1. Kierkegaard, S. (2009). *Concluding Unscientific Postscript*. A. Hannay (Trans.). London: Cambridge University Press. (Original work published in 1846.)

2. Karbelnig, A. (2021). Resuscitating the (nearly) dead profession of psychoanalysis: a review of and comment on the future of psychoanalysis: the debate about the training analyst system by Peter Zagermann. *International Journal of Controversial Discussions*, 4: 147–162.

3. Amor Towles, A. (2016). *A Gentleman in Moscow*. New York, NY: Hutchinson.

4. Hegel, G.W.F. (1977). *Phenomenology of Spirit*. Trans. A.V. Miller. Oxford: Oxford University Press. (Original work published in 1807.)

5. Mills, J. (2002). *The Unconscious Abyss; Hegels' Anticipation of Psychoanalysis.* Albany, NY: State University of New York Press, p. 192.

6. Fichte, J.G. (1794–1795/1982). *The Science of Knowledge.* P. Heath & J. Lachs (Trans.). Cambridge: Cambridge University Press.

7. Lichtenberg, J.D. (1989). *Psychoanalysis and Motivation.* New York, NY: Analytic Press.

8. Atwood, G.E., & Stolorow, R.D. (2014). *Structures of Subjectivity.* New York, NY: Routledge.

9. Galatzer-Levy, R.M. (1995). Psychoanalysis and dynamical systems theory: prediction and self similarity. *Journal of the American Psychoanalytic Association* 43: 1085–1113.

10. Gabriel, M. (2017). *I Am Not a Brain.* C. Turner (Trans.). Cambridge: Polity Press, p. 6.

11. Ibid., p. 7.

12. Shedler, J. (2010). The efficacy of psychodynamic psychotherapy. *American Psychologist*, 65: 98–109.

13. Karbelnig, A. (2014). The analyst is present: viewing the psychoanalytic process as performance art. *Psychoanalytic Psychology*, 33 (Supplement 1): 153–172. Doi: 10.1037/a0037332.

14. Lacan, J. (1960). *The Seminar of Jacques Lacan, Book IV: The Ethics of Psychoanalysis.* J.A. Miller (Ed.) & D. Porter (Trans.). New York, NY: Norton.

15. Winnicott, D.W. (1992). *Through Paediatrics to Psycho-Analysis.* New York, NY: Brunner-Routledge, p. 185.

16. Winnicott, D.W. (1965). *The Maturational Processes and the Facilitating Environment: Studies in the Theory of Emotional Development.* London: Hogarth.

17. Kohut, H. (1977). *The Restoration of the Self.* Chicago, IL: University of Chicago Press.

18. Grotstein, J.S. (1990). The contribution of attachment theory and self-regulation theory to the therapeutic alliance. *Modern Psychoanalysis*, 15(2): 169–184.

19. Linnaeus, C. (1959). *Systema Naturae: A Photographic Facsimile of the First Volume of the Tenth Edition.* London: British Museum. (Original work published in 1758.)

20. Rangell, L. (2004). *My Life in Theory.* New York, NY: JAPA Press.

21. Stepansky, P. (2009). *Psychoanalysis at the Margins.* New York, NY: Other Press.

22. Goldberg, A. (1999). *Being of Two Minds: The Vertical Split in Psychoanalysis and Psychotherapy.* Northdale, NJ: The Analytic Press.

Index